6.95

b/2

Ii0672262

HEAD INJURY IN CHILDREN AND ADOLESCENTS

A RESOURCE AND REVIEW FOR SCHOOL AND ALLIED PROFESSIONALS

SECOND EDITION

Vivian Begali

Charlottesville Public Schools
Charlottesville, Virginia

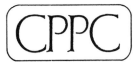

Clinical Psychology Publishing Company, Inc.
4 Conant Square
Brandon, VT 05733

Library of Congress Cataloging-in-Publication Data

Begali, Vivian.
    Head injury in children and adolescents : a resource and review for school and allied professionals / Vivian Begali. -- 2nd ed.
        p.   cm.
    Includes bibliographical references.
    ISBN 0-88422-098-2 (paper) : $29.95
    1. Brain--Wounds and injuries--Complications.   2. Brain-damaged children--Psychology.   3. Brain-damaged children--Education.
4. Brain-damaged children--Mental health.   I. Title.
    [DNLM: 1. Brain Injuries--in adolescence.   2. Brain Injuries--in infancy & childhood.   WS 340 B416h]
RJ496.B7B44   1992
617.4'81044'083--dc20
DNLM/DLC
for Library of Congress   92-52847
                                                                                        CIP

 4 Conant Square
Brandon, Vermont 05733

Cover design: Michael F. Gauthier

Printed in the United States of America.

To the survivors and their champions . . .

CONTENTS

Contents

Contents

Contents

FIGURES

ACKNOWLEDGMENTS

The second edition of any book evolves out of the first creation and carries with it the original sources of inspiration and influence. My former colleagues at the Klugé Children's Rehabilitation Center of the University of Virginia Medical Center and many well-remembered survivors of THI continue to serve as lucid reminders of the importance of spreading the word. The psychology faculty of James Madison University yet deserves my gratitude for recommending publication of the original manuscript. I also wish to acknowledge my present-day colleagues in the Charlottesville Public Schools, whose professionalism and sensibility have served as reliable tests for the recommendations and content herein. Finally, I wish to acknowledge my parents, Richard and Rose Begali, who have always been encouraging forces in my life, and my husband, Frederick Imboden, who has lovingly endured yet another bout of my preoccupation.

PREFACE

It is important for school and allied professionals to be knowledgeable about traumatic head injury (THI) and its effect upon the educational performance of children and adolescents. Any number or combination of cognitive, behavioral, and physical complications can result when the brain is damaged. Traumatic brain injury can cause mild to major personality changes, varying degrees of intellectual deterioration, disinhibited social behavior, memory loss, sensory impairment, and/or persistent motor residua. Even the mildest forms of cerebral injury can negatively impact a child's ability to concentrate, attend, process information, and remember. School performance and social functioning can be permanently altered.

By the time moderately or severely brain-injured students return to school, they are likely to have endured a lengthy and arduous hospitalization. Both survivor and family have been forced to face major life changes. Memories, experiences, dreams, and expectations may have been permanently disrupted. The THI child's return to the public schools following hospitalization generally occurs during an advanced stage of recovery. Because the brain continues to undergo substantial reorganization long after a traumatic insult, the capacity for further restoration beyond the point of school re-entry exists. The first several years following a traumatic head injury bear a concentrated potential for recovery. Consequently, those responsible for intervention cannot afford to expend this precious time casually.

Recent amendments to federal education mandates for children with disabilities are expected to influence the service offered to traumatically brain-injured students. These federal changes lend muscle to years of advocacy efforts aimed at promoting the educational needs of traumatically brain-injured children and formally confirm the distinction between THI and other disabilities. Section 602(a)(1) of the Individuals with Disabilities Education Act (formerly the Education for the Handicapped Act, PL 94-142) now designates "traumatic brain injury" as a separate category within the definition of "children with disabilities." As school professionals increase their knowledge about THI and its effects, the reflexive tendency to fit THI students into ill-suited programs for the sake of convenience or tradition will be replaced by greater flexibility and a reliance upon treatment strategies that promote, rather than compromise, recovery. Furthermore, educational teams will have at their disposal the legislative backing needed to create and implement responsive educational treatment programs – programs that reflect state-of-the-art practices in head injury rehabilitation.

The point, here, is not to equate educational systems with hospitals, nor to suggest that school systems become responsible for comprehensive clinical care. Although it is true that many of the intricacies of THI are indeed medical in nature, these intricacies impact learning and school functioning with no less intensity or significance. Many of the goals maintained by rehabilitation centers for THI patients are equally applicable and relevant for the educational setting. For example, goals related to self-management; daily living; academic, social, and vocational training; community survival; and counseling have merit across settings. As educational systems face the challenges of THI, there is little reason to overlook the vast groundwork laid in the field of head injury rehabilitation. For the most part, much of what has been proven successful in clinical settings is applicable with modification to the educational setting. Rehabilitation methods can be used to close the gap between the new and familiar.

A comprehensive view of traumatic head injury that incorporates medical, physiological, neuropsychological, rehabilitative, and behavioral dimensions puts professionals in proper position to individualize instruction and maximize recovery. This second edition has been written with this goal in mind. The contents reflect a convergence of theory, treatment, multidisciplinary influences, and personal experience. The perspectives of a number of disciplines are represented to call attention to the multidimensional, yet interactive nature of optimal service delivery following THI. In the interest of establishing a comprehensive basis by which to comprehend THI, background on etiology, epidemiology, neuropathology, treatment, outcome, long-term effects, and educational implications has been included. Personal experience in medical and educational settings as both an educator and psychologist has made the goal of providing an integrated and broad-based view of THI possible. This second edition updates and expands the coverage of *Head Injury in Children and Adolescents: A Resource and Review for School and Allied Professionals* as new research and directions have been incorporated.

Since publication of the first edition, I have had the pleasure of providing consultative services to a wide range of professionals whose questions and practical concerns about traumatic brain injury have served as the catalyst for modifications and added features to this second edition of the book. Over 600 references are included, of which approximately 150 are new. Each chapter has been revised with the intention of updating the reader on new research and trends while preserving the all important historical and multidisciplinary emphasis. It is intended that this text serve as an initial reference for school practitioners and allied professionals entering into direct service with traumatically brain-injured children and adolescents. This resource may be used as (a) the basis for further study of THI; (b) a guide for the interpretation of transdisciplinary research and terminology; (c) a reference for developing suitable educational programs and policies relevant to THI students; and (d) a source of rationale for creating original programmatic solutions to the challenges that THI brings. The contents have been arranged in a spiraling manner to provide the practitioner with a logical and progressive presentation of head injury, beginning with an integration of medical and educational parameters, definitions, acute care, epidemiology, and sequelae, and culminating in the practical issues of assessment, intervention, and program planning.

Chapter 1 sets the stage by relating THI to the educational domain and developing a framework for its conceptualization. The clinical parameters of THI are introduced in chapter 2. THI is defined and the broad classes of open and closed head injuries are distinguished according to associated primary and secondary damage and the consequences that result. The essential steps and foci of acute medical care and epidemiological data emphasize the serious nature of THI and its prevalence. The neurological and medical means for assessing severity and the prognostic differences between mild, moderate, and severe injuries are addressed in chapter 3. Chapter 4 includes a practical and basic overview of neuroanatomy and pertinent neuropsychological principles. A detailed discussion of prognosis and outcome, a description of the recovery process, and theories of brain recovery are included in chapter 5. The second section of this book, which includes chapters 6, 7, and 8, is focused on the physical, cognitive, psychiatric, and psychosocial sequelae that complicate THI and their implications for the educational setting. The formal assessment of THI individuals is discussed in chapter 9, which includes descriptions of the more popular neuropsychological batteries and a comprehensive list of supplemental assessment procedures. Guidelines for conducting, organizing, and interpreting assessment results following THI are provided. Chapter 10 outlines specific educational strategies and covers treatment rationale. Special attention is given to the fundamentals of cognitive rehabilitation (viz., academic retraining, memory therapy, language therapy, perceptual retraining); behavioral management, individual and family counseling, social skills training, and psychopharmacology. A number of case illustrations provide added insight. Chapter 11 addresses the practical matters of transition and re-entry, service delivery, and individualized program development. The appendices include descriptive information about specialized equipment, sources for organizational support and computer programs, and practical guidelines for seizure care.

V. L. Begali

1

INTRODUCTION: SETTING THE STAGE

Over the past 15 years, the chances for survival following traumatic head injury (THI) have increased due to such modern medical and technical advances as computed tomographic (CT) scanning, improved methods of intensive care, specialized shock trauma centers, and well-orchestrated emergency evacuation teams (Brinkman, 1979; Mahoney et al., 1983; Noble, Conley, Laski, & Noble, 1990). It has been estimated that between 500,000 and 750,000 new cases of traumatic head injury requiring hospitalization occur each year in the United States (Frankowski, Annegers, & Whitman, 1985; Kalsbeek, McLaurin, Harris, & Miller, 1980). The annual number of head injuries exceeds 1 million if all lacerations and contusions to the head are included in the estimates (Frankowski et al., 1985). Approximately 20–40% of all incident head injuries produce moderate to severe disability. Up to 10% are fatal. Incidence rates for school-aged children suggest that roughly 150–550 per 100,000 sustain THI yearly; approximately 90% of them survive (Frankowski et al., 1985). The majority of school-aged survivors eventually return to the public school system, many with a need for special education services (Klonoff, Low, & Clark, 1977; Rosen & Gerring, 1986).

The educational needs and distinctions of traumatically brain-injured children have long been overlooked and minimized. This oversight has resulted in the erroneous classification of THI children and adolescents as mentally retarded (MR), learning disabled (LD), or seriously emotionally disturbed (SED). Persistent advocacy efforts,

1

however, have prompted recent federal legislative action on behalf of traumatically brain-injured children. The Individuals with Disabilities Education Act (IDEA) (formerly the Education of the Handicapped Act) incorporates the Amendments of 1990 which include "traumatic brain injury" as 1 of 13 specified educational disabilities (20 U.S.C. 1401). THI children whose educational performance is adversely affected by traumatic brain injury and who, by reason thereof, need special education and related services, are now so entitled. Federal conditions of reimbursement have been imposed upon state and local educational agencies to encourage the provision of a free, appropriate public education and procedural guarantees for traumatically brain-injured children (Federal Register, 1991).

Beyond the mandate for a free, appropriate public education and the fiscal incentives imposed by Federal legislation, the incorporation of traumatic brain injury into the spectrum of educational disabilities, for the first time, formally distinguishes THI children from those whose impairment is the result of mental retardation, a specific learning disability, or serious emotional disturbance. In the years to come, this legal precedent is expected to sensitize the public to the unique consequences of brain injury and will undoubtedly influence school policy, assessment practices, instructional methodology, program implementation, and placement practices where THI children are concerned. Legislative and fiscal incentives aside, public school systems are notoriously slow to change. Established organizational procedures, endemic regulatory demands, and considerable educational responsibility encumber efficient implementation of even the most promising of educational initiatives. Knowledgeable professionals within the system, however, can effect immediate changes in the manner and extent to which THI children are served. Professionals can accelerate the process of change by developing a comprehensive understanding of the nature of brain injury, by practicing proven treatment strategies, and by leading others toward accomplishment of the same.

Until legislation is strictly enforced and THI is thoroughly understood, traumatically brain-injured children and adolescents are likely to be placed in classrooms intended for the mentally retarded, learning disabled, or seriously emotionally disturbed, and will be treated accordingly. Although it is true that some school-aged children with traumatic brain injury can be adequately served within traditional special education classrooms (or even with minor adjustments made to regular education programs), the implication that the parameters of THI are somehow similar to those of MR, LD, or SED by virtue of association should be actively challenged. Faulty assumptions will lead to superficial and biased estimates of cognitive potential, incomplete appraisals of learning needs, and a disregard for cognitive, physical, and behavioral uniqueness (Begali, 1987), in which case, federal legislation will have accomplished very little.

With many school systems now offering departmentalized or noncategorical models of special education service delivery, there is a tendency to dilute etiological distinctions among disabled children. An exclusive emphasis upon group similarities as opposed to individual differences will work against the best interests of the THI child whose continued recovery depends upon the discriminate application of proven educational and rehabilitative techniques capable of restoring or circumventing child-specific neurobehavioral dysfunction of atypical quality. If THI children continue to be served in classrooms intended for those whose cognitive, physical, emotional, and behavioral needs are significantly different, then well-informed school professionals will be the first and primary line of defense.

Certainly, many of the learning problems head-injured students experience as a group are similar to those experienced by developmentally disabled and emotionally disturbed children, namely, problems with attention, impulse control, problem solving, skill integration, abstract thinking, and social judgment (Cohen, Joyce, Rhoades, & Welks, 1985). Moreover, few would argue that head-injured pupils requiring special education are just as likely to benefit from individualized strategies and good teaching as other exceptional learners. Task analysis, multisensory approaches, compensatory training, practice and repetition, adaptive instruction, consideration of processing styles, and so forth, are sound and popular strategies routinely recommended for teaching most children with learning problems (Bush & Giles, 1969; Hallahan et al., 1983; Johnson & Myklebust, 1967; Wang, Reynolds, & Schwartz, 1989).

The real distinction between optimal programming for groups of MR, LD, or SED students and those who are THI is not simply a matter of technical finesse. More precisely, the distinction lies in the application of knowledge and principles relevant to THI and the extent to which classroom strategies are adjusted to accommodate the neuropsychological idiosyncrasies of each brain-injured child. It is the professional who must first prepare, adapt, and ultimately execute instructional strategies and treatment techniques in a manner that enhances recovery and facilitates compensation. When meeting the needs of traumatically brain-injured children, school professionals will face the challenges of atypical performance styles, unique and undulating ability profiles, irregular rates of progress, contrasting potentials for recovery, and marked within-student variability. As a group, head-injured students can be distinguished from other exceptional populations by (a) their developmental history (THI students are likely to have experienced a period of relatively uncompromised and normal development); (b) the cause of their disability and its sudden onset; (c) the range and precarious nature of their cognitive, physical, and emotional states; (d) the coexistence of associated cognitive, physical, sensory, and emotional complications; and (e) the often variable and unpredictable course of their progress (Begali, 1987).

THI students can be distinguished from the "mentally retarded." Mental retardation implies "significantly subaverage general intellectual functioning existing concurrently with deficits in adaptive behavior and manifested during the developmental period, which adversely affects a child's educational performance" (Federal Register, 1977, p. 42478). Although THI youngsters may yield subaverage IQ scores and show deficits in adaptive behavior following the injury, such deficits are often short-lived (Black, Blumer, Wellner, & Walker, 1971; Boll, 1982). On the whole, THI students have the potential to improve their intellectual standing, if not reestablish their former IQ (Boll, 1983; Klonoff et al., 1977; Levin, Eisenberg, & Miner, 1983). The same is true of their academic and adaptive behavior skills. This potential for significant improvement runs contrary to the general prognosis associated with mental retardation, wherein intellectual status (i.e., IQ) is expected to remain relatively constant and achievement profiles characteristically flat with little chance for academic skills to progress beyond the 6th-grade level (Sattler, 1982). Unlike MR, which results from biological, medical, or cultural-familial factors (Heward & Orlansky, 1980), THI occurs suddenly and is often preceded by a period of normal development and adequate intellectual functioning. On the issue of sudden late-onset intellectual subnormality due to brain injury, Robinson and Robinson (1965) made the point years ago that the label of mental retardation is inappropriate in cases wherein deficit functioning is not a carryover from earlier development. They suggested that structural or functional cause of intellectual change (e.g., traumatic head injury) be used to describe condition (i.e., traumatically brain injured).

THI students can be distinguished from the "seriously emotionally disturbed." The educational definition of seriously emotionally disturbed implies:

> (a) an inability to learn which cannot be explained by intellectual, sensory, or health factors; (b) an inability to build or maintain satisfactory interpersonal relationships with peers and teachers; (c) inappropriate types of behavior or feelings under normal circumstances; (d) a general pervasive mood of unhappiness or depression; or (e) a tendency to develop physical symptoms or fears associated with personal or school problems. (Federal Register, 1977, p. 42478)

Although THI students may exhibit problems with interpersonal relationships, inappropriate behaviors, and various disorders of affect (Benton, 1979b; Boll, 1982; Levin & Grossman, 1978; Lehr, 1990d), their problems are primarily the result of sudden neurological disruption (unless postinjury disturbances are extensions of a premorbid condition). Rutter (1981) hypothesized that the link between psychiatric consequence and brain injury is not necessarily causal. Behavioral and emotional disorders following THI may be (a) the result of stress associated with the injury, (b) a response to physical loss, (c) the result of intellectual impairment, (d) the result of psychosocial deprivation, or (e) related to the conditions that led up to the injury. Accordingly, the emotional disorders that surface subsequent to THI can be explained by psychosocial, intellectual, sensory, and/or neurological factors, which are either (a) unchanged or exacerbated by the injury, or (b) a direct consequence. In any case, THI remains the primary handicapping condition and should, therefore, serve as the criterion for instructional and placement decisions. Because of the many neuropsychological deficits to accompany THI, such as poor memory, significant problems with cause and effect relationships, difficulty reading social cues, attentional problems, and lack of foresight (Barin, Hanchett, Jacob, & Scott, 1985; Boll, 1982;

HEAD INJURY IN CHILDREN AND ADOLESCENTS

TABLE 1

DISTINGUISHING TRAUMATIC HEAD INJURY (THI) FROM SPECIFIC LEARNING DISABILITY (SLD)

THI	SLD
Onset sudden due to external event; preceded by period of normal, uncompromised development	Congenital, perinatal, or early onset
Follows loss of consciousness, hence, clear evidence of neurological damage	No coma
Marked pre-post-injury contrast in cognitive, behavioral, physical capabilities	No before-after contrast
Requires emergency medical care or extended hospitalization	Hospitalization not required
Paresis, paralysis, spasticity may result requiring specialized treatment	Physical problems generally limited to poor coordination
Mild to severe sensory perceptual impairment	Mild sensory perceptual deficits
Distractibility is provoked by internal and external stimuli	Distractibility provoked by external stimuli
Moderate to severe problems with memory and new learning	Mild memory problems
Disability can result in cognitive, sensory, motor, behavioral, and emotional complications	Disability confined to parameters of psychological processing disorder
Mild to severe speech/language problems	Mild to moderate speech/language problems
Difficulty recognizing and accepting post-injury deficits	Aware of learning deficits
Discrepancies in ability levels pronounced; some may resume preinjury status, others will remain markedly deficient; progress is rapid during early and middle stages of recovery	Discrepancies show little relative change; potential for splinter skill development is possible; progress is slow and developmentally sequenced
Emotional expressions are unpredictable and exaggerated	Emotional outbursts are generally situational in nature

(continued)

TABLE 1

(CONTINUED)

THI	SLD
Complex array of neurobehavioral complications require modified and intensive application of instructional and management techniques	Responsive to traditional instructional techniques and behavioral management strategies
Pronounced problems with reasoning, organization of thoughts, cause–effect relationships, and problem solving	Capable of independent thinking
Prone to fatigue and overstimulation; may require shortened school day or modified schedule	Capable of withstanding facets of typical school day and full course load
May require intensive vocational training program and supervised employment	Capable of achieving vocational self-sufficiency

Goethe & Levin, 1984; Levin, Benton, & Grossman, 1982; Rimel, Giordani, Barth, Boll, & Jane, 1981), THI students do not necessarily respond to traditional behavioral management strategies in the same way that non-brain-injured students with emotional disorders respond (Divack, Herrle, & Scott, 1985; Newcombe, 1981).

THI students can be distinguished from the "learning disabled." A specific learning disability is defined as:

> a disorder in one or more of the basic psychological processes involved in understanding or in using language, spoken or written, which may manifest itself in an imperfect ability to listen, think, speak, read, write, spell, or to do mathematical calculations. (Federal Register, 1977, p. 42478)

Of all the existing categorical definitions used to describe exceptional children and adolescents, THI students are most likely to be inappropriately classified as LD (NHIF, 1985). There is no question that THI students experience specific learning problems. These problems are not, however, the result of congenital or perinatal complications, biochemical imbalances, or maturational or motivational influences (Heward & Orlansky, 1980; Sattler, 1982). Although the federal definition of LD includes "brain injury" as one of its qualifying conditions, the implication is one of *minimal* brain injury due to congenital or perinatal influences. The learning deficits associated with minimal brain dysfunction are typically less dramatic than the cognitive and behavioral sequelae associated with adventitious brain injury produced by an external physical agent (Cohen et al., 1985; NHIF, 1985).

Table 1 offers a comparison between the distinguishing features of traumatic head injury (THI) and specific learning disability (SLD) (Begali, 1987; Burns & Gianutsos, 1987; Cohen et al., 1985; Lehr, 1990b; Rutter, 1981; NHIF, 1985).

Professionals who intend to treat children and adolescents with THI effectively must possess an understanding of the nature of brain injury, its consequences, and the process of recovery. Without an appreciation for the unique characteristics that set THI individuals apart, educational professionals will find it difficult to pace instruction, accomplish meaningful objectives, and structure appropriate program services (Begali, 1987; Levin & Eisenberg, 1979). Those who treat traumatically brain-injured students will need to adopt an entirely new frame of reference by which to gauge, interpret, and promote progress. The process of recovery, in general, and the phenomenon of "spontaneous recovery" or the sparing of function, in particular, are but two unique facets of traumatic brain injury. Both merit special consideration as both will influence the educational process. For the traumatically brain injured, the process of recovery carries powerful educational implications. The nuances of recovery following THI will influence the rate and extent to which progress is realized, not to mention the ways in which it is promoted and assessed. For example, it is essential to know that motor recovery following THI typically precedes cognitive recovery. In practical terms, this means that a seemingly restored physical appearance is not proof that the complex cognitive effects of brain damage have abated, i.e., that the potential for residual cognitive dysfunction exists despite normal appearances and, as such, merits careful investigation. Furthermore, "normal" test results and isolated pockets of preserved or recovered abilities can be easily misread by the unaccustomed professional as evidence of full recovery when, in fact, both are common occurrences following THI and neither is just cause for scientific optimism. It is equally important for professionals to recognize that the first several years following traumatic brain injury hold the greatest potential for change and functional restoration (Barth & Macciocchi, 1985; Kaufman et al., 1985). In practical terms this means that optimal use must be made of this critical stage, i.e., treatment efforts and assessment practices must be sensitive to rapid changes, the reemergence of discrete functions, and variable performances. One can well imagine the degree of educational mismanagement that can follow when educational teams fail to account for the distinguishing features of traumatic brain injury.

With the inclusion of traumatic brain injury as a separate category of educational disability, parents are expected to look toward the public schools for special services with increasing regularity and at earlier stages of the recovery continuum. This inevitable trend will require school personnel to become better acquainted with the theoretical underpinnings and practical aspects of head injury rehabilitation. A comprehensive and pragmatic understanding of head trauma is imperative if one is to make sense of posttraumatic behavior and to intervene with confidence and skill. Although the literature is replete with medically based data regarding the physiology and treatment of head injury in its early stages, relatively little attention has been paid to the long-term treatment of children or the role of the public school as an extension of the rehabilitative process. Legislative recognition of traumatic brain injury will undoubtedly spur an influx of child-focused and educational resources that address THI in the years ahead.

Traumatic brain injury is not a unidimensional impairment; hence, it cannot be adequately understood in unidimensional terms. It is a condition with medical, psychological, emotional, behavioral, and physical parameters. These parameters carry significant educational implications. This book addresses traumatic head injury in its broadest context. Research from the disciplines of pediatric medicine, neurology, neuropsychology, special education, physical and occupational therapy, rehabilitative medicine, speech/language pathology, psychology, and social work has been incorporated throughout the chapters to follow, in order to provide practitioners with a comprehensive and multidisciplinary view of THI.

2

TRAUMATIC HEAD INJURY: ESTABLISHING THE PARAMETERS

What Is Traumatic Head Injury?

Differences in the way head injury is regarded abound in the literature. Given the many treatment specialists involved at successive points along the postinjury continuum, it is reasonable to expect that such variables as degree of impairment, prognosis for recovery, and goals of treatment will undergo frequent revision and be subject to various schemes of interpretation. Neurosurgeons who deal with head injury in its acute stages view the effects of head trauma from a neuropathological perspective. Rehabilitation specialists aim to restore functional independence with the ultimate goal of community reintegration. Public school professionals will judge head injury by the way it affects educational capability.

Head injury is first and formally diagnosed by a physician on the basis of routine observation, neurological examination, and accident history (Bakay & Glasauer, 1980). Nevertheless, the criteria for what constitutes head injury are not uniform. Definitions of traumatic head injury vary among and within medical and allied professions. Some medical definitions of head injury include cases of minor facial laceration, jaw fractures, and nose injuries, even though brain dysfunction is not suspected (World Health Organization [WHO], 1975). Others require that an alteration in consciousness or evidence of neurological deficit prevail. Some descriptions of head injury have been developed to reflect admission policies at various hospitals and treatment centers (Jennett & Teasdale, 1981). Still others have

10

been customized to accommodate the design of experimental studies.

The International Classification of Diseases-Ninth Revision (ICD-9) (1986) is the basis of official statistics on various pathologies and is generally regarded as a diagnostic index of sorts. In the case of head injury, however, the ICD-9 offers a set of ten rubrics pertaining to head injuries which are neither mutually exclusive nor useful, according to Jennett and Teasdale (1981). The rubrics are seldom relied upon in the literature and are inconsistently applied. For example, the same injury using ICD-9 rubrics might be termed "concussion," "injury unspecified," or "unqualified skull fracture," depending upon local custom (Jennett & Teasdale, 1981). This system is not ranked to adequately reflect the severity of the injury (Levin, Benton, & Grossman, 1982). Moreover, the external cause of the injury, with the exception of "motor vehicle accident," is not specifiable. While such ICD-9 terms as "concussion," "contusion," and "fracture" convey some meaning, they are of limited practical advantage when attempting to formulate a prognosis for recovery or project goals of treatment.

More insight into the nature of an injury and its potential consequences can be generated from a knowledge of the causal agent (Meirowsky, 1984; Pang, 1985) and the nature, extent, and site of the damage (Rourke, Bakker, Fisk, & Strang, 1983). For example, it is potentially more useful to know whether an injury is open (the result of a penetrating injury, likely to cause localized brain damage about the path of the object) or closed (probably the result of an acceleration/deceleration injury, likely to cause diffuse damage), and whether the injury is considered mild, moderate, or severe (each degree of severity being associated with a general prognosis for recovery and probable sequelae). Further insight into the consequences of THI may be gained from knowing whether significant brain damage has occurred to the right versus left hemisphere, frontal versus temporal lobe, or brain stem versus cortex (Lezak, 1983; Luria, 1963; Rourke et al., 1983). [Discussion of these and other determinants pertinent to the understanding of outcome following head injury will be resumed subsequently and in forthcoming chapters.]

The National Head Injury Foundation (1988) refers to head injury as a traumatic insult to the brain capable of producing physical, intellectual, emotional, social, and vocational changes. This definition of head injury implies brain damage and associated dysfunction. It is the dysfunction caused by brain damage that poses a concern to school and rehabilitative personnel; brain damage can compromise the ability to coordinate movements, speak, reason, or mediate behavior. The fundamental goal of educational programming and rehabilitative treatment is to promote recovery from brain damage by remediating dysfunction and/or compensating for its effects (Jennett & Teasdale, 1981; Luria, 1963).

For purposes of this text, the term *traumatic head injury* implies mild to severe adventitious brain damage and associated dysfunction. Specifically, a traumatic head injury is defined as the product of a definite physical blow or wound to the head that is significant enough to produce (a) an alteration in consciousness, no matter how brief, and/or (b) associated neurological or neurobehavioral dysfunction. *Not included* in this definition are cases of facial laceration, lower jaw fractures, trauma to the eye, ear, or nose (unless the aforementioned criteria are otherwise met), or injuries associated with birth trauma. The term traumatic head injury is used synonymously with traumatic brain injury, cerebral injury, craniocerebral trauma, head trauma, and traumatic cerebral injury.

It should be noted that there are, of course, other causes of brain damage besides physical injury to the head, although they are not intended to be the focus of this text. To help the reader place THI into perspective, other possible causes of brain damage are metabolic dysfunction, toxicity, degenerative brain disease, hereditary disease, cerebral vascular disease, convulsive disorders, fetal and birth injury, and tumors (Bakay & Glasauer, 1980; Fenichel, 1988; Sattler, 1982).

Classes of Traumatic Head Injury

Brain damage as a result of THI refers to a structural or physiological change in the nerve tissue of the brain to a pathological degree (Sattler, 1982). North (1984) specifically attributes brain damage from head injury to (a) structural lesions directly caused by the impact (primary damage); (b) secondary damage due to raised intracranial pressure, brain swelling, infection, hemorrhage, and oxygen deprivation (hypoxia); and (c) metabolic changes such a hyperthermia (excessive fever), electrolyte disturbances (salt and water retention), damage to the hypothalamus or pituitary gland, and hyperventilation (increased respiration).

There are two major classes of THI, namely, open and closed. Open (penetrating) head injuries typically produce discrete and focal lesions. Closed head injuries tend to cause generalized or diffuse cerebral involvement.

Open Head Injury. Traumatic head injury that results when the scalp and/or skull is penetrated, as in a gunshot or missile wound, is an open head injury (Bakay & Glasauer, 1980; Lezak, 1983; Meirowsky, 1984). The agents commonly responsible for open craniocerebral injuries are bullets, rocks, shell fragments, knives, and blunt instruments. Primary brain damage due to an open head injury tends to be localized about the path of the penetrating object, as in a stab or bullet wound (Cooper, 1982). Primary damage may also occur from penetrating bone fragments or shattered pieces of shells or bullets (Levin, Benton, & Grossman, 1982). Surgical cleansing of the wounds (debridement) removes most of the damaged tissue often leaving the remainder of the brain spared and uncompromised (Cooper, 1982; Lezak, 1983; Meirowsky, 1984). High velocity missiles, commonly seen in wartime injuries, can produce other remote lesions as a result of the missile's displacement forces which push the brain surface against the skull. These lesions are similar to those seen in closed head injuries and are most often detected at the base of the brain (Shapiro, 1983). Low velocity projectiles, such as bullets which do not sustain enough energy to exit the skull, may produce additional damage as they ricochet off the skull while continuing to traverse the brain (Bakay & Glasauer, 1980; Shapiro, 1983).

In addition to the direct (primary) damage, a penetrating injury may also produce secondary damage throughout the brain as a result of intracranial pressure effects, swelling, bleeding (Cooper, 1982; Lezak, 1983), and cranial and intracranial infection (Cooper, 1982; Meirowksy, 1984; Rutter, Chadwick, & Shaffer, 1983). Unlike closed head injury, open head injuries rarely lead to coma, but the risk of epilepsy is much greater (Jennett, 1975a; Lishman, 1978). Between 17% and 43% of all patients with open head injury develop seizures (Levin, Benton, & Grossman, 1982) compared with 5% in the closed head injury population (Jennett, 1979).

Because the major lesions of open head injuries are usually focalized (confined), the intellectual losses due to damage are relatively circumscribed and predictable (Lezak, 1983). In addition to the specific intellectual and behavior changes that correspond with the original site of lesion, open head injuries may result in memory impairment, mental slowing, problems with attention and concentration, and changes in the ability to deal with everyday intellectual demands (Lezak, 1983).

In a follow-up study (Kaufman et al., 1985), the quality of long-term outcome following civilian gunshot wounds to the head was assessed in six survivors (four adults and two children) at 1 year post injury. Deficits in long-term memory for new information were the most common sequelae. The presence of linguistic versus visual-spatial deficits was related to laterality, that is, the hemisphere affected. Specifically, visual-spatial deficits were consistent with right-sided lesions as were mild word-finding difficulties. Left-hemisphere lesions produced receptive and expressive language aberrations. Both children (aged 9 and 11 years) required special education placement upon their return to school because of associated cognitive and behavioral disturbances (viz., withdrawal, distractibility, extreme dependency).

Persons who sustain an open head injury tend to make relatively rapid gains during the first 2 years following injury, with further improvement occurring in subsequent years in some, but not necessarily all areas of deficit (Kaufman et al., 1985). Language and constructional disorders are among other functions that tend to improve (Lezak, 1983), whereas localized sensory deficits (e.g., visual impairment, visual field deficits, reduced tactile sensitivity) and distractibility are prone to persist (Kampen & Grafman, 1989; Teuber, 1974).

Closed Head Injury. Two distinctive mechanical factors have been identified as producing brain damage in closed head injury, namely, *direct contact forces* and *inertial forces* (Alexander, 1984; Pang, 1985). Closed head injuries may or may not produce a skull fracture. The direct contact force or force of impact is the primary cause of brain damage in static injuries whereby a relatively stationary victim sustains a blow to the head (see Figure 1). Damage results from the inward compression of the skull at the point of impact, the

FIGURE 1

BRAIN DAMAGE CAUSED BY CLOSED HEAD INJURY

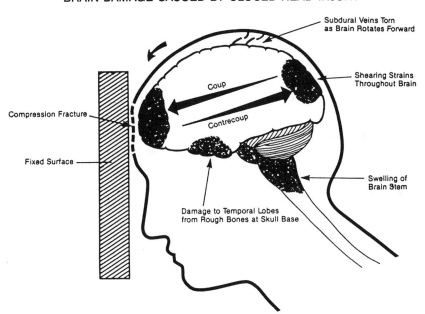

compensatory adjacent outbending that follows, and rebound effects (Lezak, 1983; Pang, 1985). The point of original impact is referred to as the *coup*; the cerebral area opposite the blow is the *contrecoup* (also *contracoup*). Contrecoup damage results from the translation of force and the direction of impact to the brain. The force of the blow may literally bounce the brain off the opposite side of its bony container, bruising brain tissue where it strikes the skull (Levin, Benton, & Grossman, 1982; Lezak, 1983). Both coup and contrecoup lesions account for the specific and localizable behavioral alterations that accompany closed head injury (Lezak, 1983).

Inertial forces at play in motor vehicle accidents (acceleration/ deceleration injuries) generate other types of injury. First, the continuation of brain movement and rotation within the skull following surface contact puts strain on delicate nerve fibers and blood vessels which can cause shearing (Langfitt & Gennarelli, 1982; Strich, 1969). Coma results from a disruption of the nerve fibers or, more specifically, severe diffuse axonal injury of the brain stem

15

reticular formation (Alexander, 1984). Severe distortions within the brain may cause instant death (Alexander, 1984; Jennett & Teasdale, 1981; Parker, 1990). Secondly, as brain surfaces are pushed against the inner surface of the skull upon sudden deceleration, the brain sustains bruising (contusions). Focal cortical contusions caused by inertial impact against the dense irregularities of the skull generally result in damage to specific and predisposed regions. These lesions most often occur to the undersides of the frontal and temporal lobes (Alexander, 1984; Levin et al., 1985; Levin, 1990), the consequences of which are likely to involve behavior, affect, emotions, memory, and attention (Alexander, 1984). In addition to the direct physiological consequences of closed head injury, secondary phenomena such as brain swelling, elevated intracranial pressure, brain shifting (herniation), infection, and unusual bleeding may ensue (Jellinger, 1983; Ransohoff & Koslow, 1978; Shapiro, 1983).

Medical Responses to THI

Treatment of Secondary Complications

As previously noted, trauma to the head, whether from open or closed injury, can produce both primary (impact damage) and secondary complications. Primary injury occurs immediately following the impact as a result of tissue disruption directly caused by the blow (Pang, 1985). Drugs and physiological manipulation are ineffectual in reversing the effects of direct and permanent tissue damage (North, 1984). Extensive primary injury, therefore, produces irreversible damage, regardless of medical or rehabilitative therapy (North, 1984; Pang, 1985; Rosen & Gerring, 1986).

The secondary damage that develops after the insult is potentially reversible with proper emergency medical care (North, 1984). Secondary complications are most often the result of (a) raised intracranial pressure; (b) infarction (death of tissue due to regional blood deprivation); (c) hypoxia (oxygen deprivation); (d) hematomas (bleeding or clotting within the skull); (e) edema (brain swelling due to an increase in its fluid content); (f) hemorrhage (rupture of cortical veins); and/or (g) infection (Friedman, 1983; Jennett & Teasdale, 1981; Levin, Benton, & Grossman, 1982; Pang, 1985). In addition, significant metabolic/hypoxic changes can occur to produce functional disturbances such as rapid and inefficient respiration and possible circulatory failure (North, 1984). Pituitary disorders arising from damage to the hypothalamus and pituitary gland, electrolyte disturbances, and/or hyperventilation may also develop (Levin, Benton, & Grossman, 1982; North, 1984; Pang, 1985).

The fundamental aim in the medical management of the secondary effects of head injury is to maintain the intracranial environment in as near normal a state as possible (Bakay & Glasauer, 1980; Shapiro, 1983). An adequate oxygen supply to the brain and metabolic rate must be maintained in order to sustain membrane potentials, electrochemical balance, the neurochemical processes responsible for synaptic transmission, and the integrity of intracellular organelles and membranes (Jennett & Teasdale, 1981). If energy to the brain, which is almost entirely produced by the oxidative metabolism of glucose in the blood, fails completely, the consequences are rapid and dramatic (Bruce, 1983). Neuronal function can fail after a matter of seconds followed by permanent structural damage within minutes (Jennett & Teasdale, 1981). Physiological manipulation (regulation of vital functions, replenishment of blood volume and nutrients, regulation of intracranial pressure), drug treatments (e.g., anticonvulsants, muscle relaxants, anesthetic agents), and surgical management (evacuation of intracranial hematomas, repair of skull fractures) may be required to minimize secondary complications (Bakay & Glasauer, 1980; North, 1984; Pang, 1985; Tabaddor, 1982).

Emergency Medical Care

When a THI child or adolescent arrives in the emergency room, a series of medical procedures are set in motion (Bakay & Glasauer, 1980). The following sequence takes the reader through the essential steps of emergency medical treatment.

1. Adequate airway and ventilation are established by means of tracheostomy, nasogastric tubes, or endotracheal intubation with mechanical ventilation; blood gas levels are monitored, and abnormalities such as increased cerebral arterial blood flow or deficient blood oxygenation are corrected.
2. Vital signs (e.g., blood pressure, heart rate) are assessed and monitored.
3. Associated injuries such as skull fractures, unusual bleeding, or internal injuries are diagnosed.

4. Level of consciousness [see Glasgow Coma Scale, chapter 3] is assessed.

5. Pupillary reflexes, visual responses, motor movements, etc., are assessed to determine neurologic status.

6. History of trauma (causal agent, duration of unconsciousness), prior seizures, medication, etc., is taken.

7. Diagnostic procedures are conducted such as computed tomography (CT) scans to locate fractures, hematomas, brain swelling, evidence of foreign bodies, and ventricular abnormalities; angiography to pinpoint vascular disorders; roentgenograms for depressed skull fractures and cervical spine injuries.

8. Medical treatment such as blood or fluid replacement, electrolyte balance, reduction of intracranial pressure and fever, and anticonvulsant therapy is provided.

9. Surgical treatment such as the cleansing and repair of scalp wounds and fractures, and the evacuation of acute hematomas, is conducted.

10. Intensive care for the severely injured is provided to include: constant monitoring and control of blood pressure, pulse, temperature, respiration, intracranial pressure; charting of vital signs and state of consciousness; care of multiple injuries; serial CT scans to detect the development of hydrocephalus, swelling, ventricular abnormalities, and lesion resolution.

Medical and Technological Advances

A growing body of experimental and clinical evidence collected from national surveys on recovery and outcome, international data banks, and autopsied head injury fatalities has permitted a more consistent application of effective treatment strategies and better patient care (Jennett & Teasdale, 1981). Modernized methods of intensive care (metabolic monitoring, drug therapy, neurosurgical methods), the development of specialized trauma centers, a growing number of better informed neurosurgical specialists, and well-staffed emergency evacuation teams have collectively contributed toward increased survival from severe head injury (Cooper, 1982; Jennett & Teasdale, 1981; Levin, Benton, & Grossman, 1982; Mahoney et al., 1983).

Computed Tomographic (CT) Scanning. With its diagnostic capability, computed tomographic (CT) scanning, in particular, has greatly advanced patient care and helped to decrease mortality (Ambrose, Gooding, & Uttley, 1976; Bakay & Glasauer, 1980; Cartlidge & Shaw, 1981). This modern noninvasive brain-imaging technique capable of producing three-dimensional images of brain tissue in the form of cross-sectional "slices" makes it possible to detect intracranial conditions (Bakay & Glasauer, 1980; Shapiro, 1983). CT scan images depict various intracranial phenomena using a density scale ranging from 0 for water (black) to 500+ for bone (white). Accordingly, clotted blood projects an image of greater density than normal brain, whereas edema and infarcted brain project as less dense (Jennett & Teasdale, 1981). CT scanning permits detection of intracranial hematomas, edema, focalized lesions, fracture sites, brain shifts, and ventricular enlargement. As a diagnostic tool, the CT scanner permits the precise and timely delivery of medical, surgical, and pharmacological interventions that help counter the secondary effects of traumatic brain injury (Bakay & Glasauer, 1980; Brink, Imbus, & Woo-Sam, 1980).

While CT scanning has all but eliminated older, more intrusive and relatively less reliable diagnostic methods (e.g., angiography, lumbar puncture, ventriculography), it too has its limitations (Cooper, 1982; North, 1984). For example, it is sometimes difficult to distinguish hematomas from normal brain tissue by means of a CT scan. In order to enhance this distinction between normal and abnormal tissue, intravenous injections of iodine contrast compounds are administered (Cooper, 1982; Jennett & Teasdale, 1981). The widespread cortical and subcortical shearing lesions, mild anterior frontal and temporal lobe lesions, and brain stem hemorrhages, however, can elude detection by CT scan despite contrast enhancement (Bakay & Glasauer, 1980; Baxter, Cohen, & Ylvisaker, 1985; Levin et al., 1985). Such lesions, although sufficiently microscopic in proportion to escape visualization by CT scan, may be significant enough to compromise a child's endurance, memory, attention, and processing abilities (Baxter et al., 1985; Boll, 1982).

School psychologists, counselors, teachers, and parents need to be aware that sophisticated medical-neurological instruments such as the CT scan and its forerunners may be unable to detect the physiological basis of mild injury, even though the child's behavior, affect, and academic performance are showing its effects (Boll, 1983; Rimel, Giordani, Barth, Boll, & Jane, 1981). Moreover, CT scans taken during the acute stages of injury often fail to detect early signs of later developing complications such as brain tissue atrophy (infarct), hydrocephalus, ventricular enlargement, and chronic sub-dural hematomas (Levin, Benton, & Grossman, 1982; Shapiro, 1983). Although the value of repeated (serial) CT scanning in detecting signs of potential lesions has been well established, this preven-tative measure is not always taken (Jennett & Teasdale, 1981). It is the astute school professional who remains vigilant for signs of possible deterioration in head-injured students and is prepared to inform parents and appropriate medical personnel of significant neurobehavioral changes.

Positron Emission Tomography (PET) Scanning. Another brain imaging technique called positron emission tomography (PET) makes it possible to locate areas of specific brain functions, pinpoint the origins of seizures, and evaluate brain tumors. The fundamen-tal principle underlying PET scanning is that chemical activity in the brain is fueled by glucose. By tracing the path of glucose within the brain, the PET scanner is able to follow the route of brain cell activity and locate sites of increased intensity. A correspondence between site of brain activity and behavioral function can be visually documented (NHIF, 1984). PET makes it possible to measure specific variables such as local cerebral metabolism and blood flow which are not measured by CT scanning. Both PET and CT scans employ ionizing forms of radiation, the cumulative effects of which may be hazardous (National Institutes of Health [NIH], 1982).

Magnetic Resonance Imaging (MRI). Recently, magnetic resonance imaging (MRI) has assumed a position of prominence in the investi-gations of brain injury among other pathological conditions (Margulis & Fisher, 1985). Relatively few disadvantages (the primary one being cost of purchase and installation), and many of the advantages of computed and positron emission tomography, make magnetic resonance imaging the research and diagnostic tool of choice (Margulis & Fisher, 1985). MRI outperforms all other imag-ing modalities without the use of ionizing radiation (Yokota,

Kurokawa, Otsuka, Kobayashi, & Nakazawa, 1991). Microscopic shearing lesions, thin subdural hematomas, degenerative processes, edema, atrophic changes, and specific white matter lesions undetected by radiographic scanning can be directly visualized by MRI (Godersky, Gentry, Trandel, Dyste, & Danks, 1990; Levin et al., 1990). Reconstructed computer images of the brain via MRI are made possible by its sensitivity to the magnetic properties of atoms in living tissue. The technique is sensitive enough to locate microscopic cell changes that heretofore had gone undetected (NHIF, 1984). MRI makes it possible to document the neuroanatomic localization of lesions associated with specific neurobehavioral consequences never before recognized by radiological technologies (Haller, Miller-Meeks, & Kardon, 1990; Levin et al., 1985; Maxwell et al., 1990).

Epidemiology

Epidemiology is the scientific study of incidence (number of new cases over a specified period of time) and patterns of distribution. Prevalence estimates are determined on the basis of carefully conducted, random surveys of the population under study or they are derived from formulas based upon incidence rates, anticipated course of disability, and the estimated life span of the sample under study. Prevalence data are useful for planning long-term residential, public school, and community programs.

Traumatic head injuries are among the most common forms of brain damage in children and young adults (Lezak, 1983). Increased mechanization and violence in our society have added to the complicated nature of THI while perpetuating its occurrence (Stover & Zeiger, 1976). Research on the cost of treatment and the complexity of head injury rehabilitation indicates its dimensions to be greater than that of any other disability group (Willer, Abosch, & Dahmer, 1990). As a result of technological and medical advances, the chances for survival following THI have improved. An estimated 88% to 95% of those who survive THI will return home following a period of treatment (Axelrod, 1986; Fife, Faich, Hollingshead, & Boynton, 1986; Kraus et al., 1984). Consequently, a significant proportion of school-aged survivors will require extraordinary effort and energy from the families, schools, and communities left to assume responsibility for their care.

Just how many school-aged children and adolescents sustain head injuries per year in the United States? How do these injuries occur and in what proportions? Precise data on the incidence, distribution, and prevalence of head injury in the United States have been difficult to ascertain. Hospital discharge surveys; patient lists from medical care providers, clinics, outpatient departments, rehabilitation centers; and household surveys have served as the primary sources of such data (Kraus, 1980).

The most frequently quoted incidence rates for head injury in the United States are taken from the National Head and Spinal Cord Injury Survey (NHSCIS) conducted by the National Institute of Neurological Disorders and Stroke of the U.S. Department of Health and Human Services (Kalsbeek et al., 1980). This descriptive epidemiological study of head trauma in the United States civilian population was the first of its kind. It remains the most frequently quoted investigation conducted. The study determined an average head injury incidence rate of 200 per 100,000. Incidence rates approximate 150 per 100,000 in children between the ages of 0–4, increasing to 550 per 100,000 between the ages of 15–24. Approximately 500,000 to 750,000 new cases of head injury requiring hospitalization are believed to occur annually. Between 30% and 50% of these injuries are moderate, severe, or fatal.

The National Health Interview Survey (NHIS), conducted two years after the NHSCIS, recorded a shocking 7,560,000 head injuries in one year. In striking contrast to the NHSCIS, this figure indicates an incidence rate of 3,486 per 100,000 (Caveness, 1979). Although a household survey such as the NHIS has the advantage of uncovering cases of head trauma that do not come to the attention of medical personnel, clinical confirmation of the diagnosis cannot be guaranteed. A 1990 report by Willer et al. on the incidence of brain injury suggests a rate of between 6 and 41 per 100,000. This statistic is by far the most conservative estimate of incidence to date because, unlike the National Health Interview Survey, its figures are based upon incidence of disability at the time of discharge rather than upon admission. Moreover, it excludes those who die at the scene and those whose injuries produce little or no neurobehavioral consequences.

Clearly, discrepancies exist among epidemiological surveys. Incidence and prevalence studies are plagued by methodological weaknesses and incongruity and, as such, obscure meaningful comparisons. A host of variables account for the disparity among figures. Failure to classify patients with head injury in a standard way, the inclusion or exclusion of persons who die at the scene or in the emergency room, and multiple counting of the same person upon hospital readmission and outpatient follow-up visits have perpetuated the problems of misclassification and misrepresentation (Kraus, 1980, 1989). Consensus does seem to prevail, however, with respect to distribution patterns. Head injury has been found to occur most often in the 15- to 24-year age group, though it is nearly as frequent in persons under the age of 15. The rate of occurrence of head injury in males is more than twice that of females. Overall, males tend to sustain more severe injuries than females. Frankowski et al. (1985) report a male to female mortality ratio of 4:1. The most common cause of head injury is motor vehicle accidents. Falls are the second most common cause of THI and the most frequent cause of mild injury in the under 15 group (Frankowski et al., 1985; Kalsbeek et al., 1980). Areas of high urban density or low socioeconomic status typically show higher incidence rates among minority populations (Frankowski et al., 1975; Jagger, Levine, Jane, & Rimel, 1984; Willer et al., 1990). When numbers are adjusted according to population ratios, no differences between the occurrence in Whites and non-Whites are evident (Kalsbeek et al., 1980).

Given the Kalsbeek et al. (1980) statistics, the average urban school district serving 10,000 students might expect as many as 20 children and adolescents per year to experience mild, moderate, or severe head injury. Certainly, not all of these students will require specialized educational provisions. Those who do, however, are likely to require extraordinary professional time and energy. Savage (1991) estimates that 1 out of every 25 students will experience some form of head trauma by the time they graduate from high school. As many as 8% to 20% of all special education students are believed to have sustained a traumatic brain injury that predates their eligibility for special education services. Despite its significance, early THI is often overlooked as a possible basis for educational problems. Given these rough estimates, it is reasonable to suspect that the educational parameters of an alarming number of traumatically brain-injured students have long been misrepresented.

HEAD INJURY IN CHILDREN AND ADOLESCENTS

Epidemiological research has demonstrated that certain factors seem to predispose age-specific populations to head injury. Alcohol consumption has been strongly implicated as a precursor to brain injury caused by motor vehicle accidents in adolescents and adults. Other less overt epidemiological factors have been associated with the incidence of head injury among school-aged children, such as premorbid psychological disorders, learning disabilities, previous head injury, juvenile delinquency, and familial discord (Naugle, 1990; Sims, 1985).

3

TRAUMATIC HEAD INJURY: ASSESSING SEVERITY

Both coma and post traumatic amnesia (PTA) are used to classify head injuries as *mild, moderate,* or *severe* (Jennett, 1975b; Jennett & Teasdale, 1981; Lishman, 1978; Russell, 1932). *Coma* is the period of unconsciousness or unawareness following brain injury (Alexander, 1984; Jennett & Teasdale, 1981; Symonds, 1962). The Head Injury Committee of the World Federation of Neurosurgical Societies has defined coma as "an unarousable, unresponsive state regardless of duration; eyes continuously closed" (Frowein, 1976). Accordingly, coma implies an absence of motor response and speech. Jennett and Teasdale (1981) argue, however, that comatose patients may be able to respond motorically to painful stimuli and show pupillary reactions and eye reflexes, and hence, prefer to view coma as "not obeying commands, not uttering words and not opening the eyes" (1981, p. 80). *Post traumatic amnesia* (PTA) includes the period of coma and extends until the patient's memory for ongoing events becomes reliable, consistent, and accurate (Alexander, 1984; Brooks, 1976; Jennett, 1975b; Russell, 1932), or, put another way, until the patient can remember today what happened yesterday (Jennett & Teasdale, 1981). A Lancet editorial (1961) originally referred to duration of PTA as the "best yardstick" available for assessing the severity of an injury. Experts continue to rely upon duration of PTA as an index of severity and consider it an equally useful prognostic indicator (Chadwick, Rutter, Shaffer, & Shrout, 1981; Levin, Benton, & Grossman, 1982; Kampen & Grafmen, 1989; Rimel, Giordani, Barth, & Jane, 1982; Russell, 1971). In addition to being able to detect the resolution of PTA upon evidence of the patient's capacity for continuous memory, its duration may be assessed retrospectively from the patient's own account of when memory was regained (Jennett & Teasdale, 1981).

Depth and duration of coma and PTA offer useful information about the severity of an injury. Depth of coma and PTA have been proven reliable gauges for predicting outcome (Frankowski et al., 1985; Levin, Benton, & Grossman, 1982; Narayan, Greenberg, Miller, & Enas, 1981; Rimel et al., 1982; Russell, 1971). Both coma and PTA offer a means by which to interpret, measure, and relay medical and neurological findings. As indexes, they are used to estimate the extent of physiological disruption present following traumatic head injury. Medical professionals have not yet agreed upon the best index for classifying injuries and predicting outcome. Until consensus is reached, the literature is likely to make reference to depth of coma, duration of coma, PTA, and others when assessing severity and predicting outcome. Early intracranial pressure (ICP) data, pupillary responses, multimodality evoked potentials (MEPs), ventricular size, and brain stem reflexes have also proven useful early predictors of outcome (Davis & Cunningham, 1984; Levin, Meyers, Grossman, & Sarwar, 1981; Narayan, Kishore, & Becker, 1982). The use of any one index as the exclusive predictor of long-term outcome is unsupported as other variables such as age, causal agent, extent of damage, site of injury, premorbid characteristics, and quality of rehabilitation interact to influence outcome (Golden, 1981a; Luria, 1963; Rourke et al., 1983; Rutter et al., 1983). Further discussion of these neurological determinants will be resumed in chapter 5. A description of two coma scales and PTA follows.

Coma Scales

The Glasgow Coma Scale (GCS) is routinely used to measure depth of coma and the severity of an injury by grading eye, motor, and verbal responses within 24 hours of the trauma (Teasdale & Jennett, 1974). In addition to its use as an index of severity, the GCS allows for the periodic monitoring of change during the early stages of recovery (Jennett & Teasdale, 1981). The GCS was originally developed to make the continuous monitoring of change in brain functioning a more systematic and reliable process within the hospital setting (Jennett, 1979).

Given that coma may be defined as unconsciousness, that is, the inability to open eyes, obey commands, or speak, the GCS makes it possible to rate such responses (or lack thereof) on a scale from 3 to 15. Conscious patients earn the highest scores. Research indicates that 90% of those with scores of 8 or less are in coma, whereas patients capable of earning scores of 9 or more are not (Rosenthal, Griffith, Bond, & Miller, 1983). Eye, motor, and verbal abilities are rated and summed according to set criteria (see Table 2). The sum is then applied to the classification scheme shown in Table 3. For the original score to be valid it must be maintained for a minimum of 6 hours from the point of impact (Rosenthal et al., 1983). Thereafter, the GCS score is used to measure change in a patient's acute condition.

1. *Eye opening.* Failure to open the eyes or to do so only in response to pain is a feature of coma. Spontaneous or noise-induced eye opening, which occurs normally, is what differentiates coma from sleep (Cartlidge & Shaw, 1981).

TABLE 2

GLASGOW COMA SCALE

Eye opening (E)	
Spontaneous	4
To speech	3
To pain	2
No response	1
Best motor response (M)	
Follows commands	6
Localization of pain	5
Withdrawal from pain	4
Flexion to pain	3
Extension to pain	2
No response	1
Verbal response (V)	
Oriented	5
Confused conversation	4
Inappropriate words	3
Incomprehensible sounds	2
No response	1

Coma Score = E + M + V

TABLE 3

CLASSIFICATION OF GLASGOW COMA SCALE TOTALS

Sum of patient responses	Degree of severity
13–15	Mild
9–12	Moderate
3–8	Severe

2. *Motor response.* The upper limbs, which generally show a greater range of movement than the lower limbs, are used to assess a motor response. In the event a patient offers more than one type of response during the course of a single examination (e.g., multiple responses by one limb, abnormality in one limb due to hemiplegia), the least abnormal or "best motor response" is used (Jennett & Teasdale, 1981).

3. *Verbal performance.* Speech is classified as oriented (normal), confused, inappropriate, incomprehensible (grunts, groans), or absent. The capacity to speak even a few words is indicative of a high level of brain functioning, although the converse is not true (Jennett & Teasdale, 1981). The absence of a verbal response during the early stages of recovery does not necessarily indicate a significant loss of cortical functioning as a verbal response may be inhibited because of an endotracheal tube, aphasia (Cartlidge & Shaw, 1981), or anxiety (Jennett & Teasdale, 1981).

Although the GCS does well to define the severity of the injury and distinguish between patients with indices of 3 versus 15, it does not necessarily follow that the long-range outcomes of these two groups will significantly differ (Rimel et al., 1981). Hence, the GCS offers critical immediate benefits, but limited prognostic utility. When applied to preverbal children, the GCS lacks reliability because the presentation of coma in young children is different from that found in adults (Lehr, 1990c).

In response to the need for a more accurate measure of early recovery in young children, Raimondi and Hirschauer (1984) developed the Children's Coma Scale (CCS) to assess consciousness in infants and children under the age of 3 (see Table 4). Due to its relatively new

TABLE 4

CHILDREN'S COMA SCALE

Ocular response (O)

Pursuit	4
Extraocular muscles intact, reactive pupils	3
Fixed pupils or extraocular muscles impaired	2
Fixed pupils and extraocular muscles paralyzed	1

Verbal response (V)

Cries	3
Spontaneous respirations	2
Apneic	1

Motor response (M)

Flexes and extends	4
Withdraws from painful stimuli	3
Hypertonic	2
Flaccid	1

Coma Score = O + V + M

status, the predictive validity of the CCS is unknown. Although the verbal response portion of the CCS is better suited for the preverbal child, its reliance upon physiological indicators may not be as accurate an index as the stimulation approach required for the GCS. The CCS uses a scale of 3 to 11 to rate the presence (or absence) of physiological indicators, whereas the GCS uses a scale of 3 to 15 to rate a patient's response to various forms of stimulation. This grading and procedural distinction restricts meaningful interscore comparisons. Furthermore, scores from the CCS cannot be applied to the classification scale used with the Glasgow Coma Scale to rank severity.

Post Traumatic Amnesia

Russell (1932) attempted to classify diffuse brain damage due to acceleration/deceleration injuries according to the length of post traumatic amnesia. Russell's classes of injury by length of PTA are as follows:

PTA less than 1 hour	–	Mild
1–24 hours	–	Moderate
1–7 days	–	Severe
Greater than 7 days	–	Very Severe

Jennett and Teasdale (1981) offer a formula for understanding the relationship between the return of speech and the end of PTA: The interval from injury to the end of PTA is approximately four times longer than the interval during which speech is absent (unless the return of speech is delayed because of aphasia, anxiety, or physical obstruction).

Lishman (1978) used length of PTA to compare cognitive loss and the ability to return to work in a study of adult patients. The generalizability of the results of this study to the outcomes in children is tenuous at best. Its use as a rough estimate of school re-entry potential in adolescents (those over 12 years of age) may, however, be somewhat predictive. Lishman determined that those whose PTAs were (a) less than 1 hour (mild injury) returned to work within 1 month; (b) between 1 hour and 24 hours (moderate) returned to work within 2 months; (c) beyond 24 hours but less than 1 week (severe) returned within 4 months; (d) greater than 1 week (very severe) were unable to return to work for at least 1 year; and (e) beyond 2 weeks were severely physically disabled, exhibited significant cognitive loss, and were not expected to work again.

Grades of Injury

When school personnel are faced with the challenge of reintegrating a head-injured student, what should be expected? How do mild, moderate, and severe injuries differ? What cognitive, behavioral, and emotional residua should be anticipated?

Mild Head Injury

Head injuries that result in a loss of consciousness or PTA of less than 1 hour (GCS 13–15) are considered mild. It has been estimated that between 50% and 75% of all traumatic head injuries are mild (Frankowski et al., 1985; Langfitt & Gennarelli, 1982). Approximately 290,000 people are hospitalized annually for mild head injuries

(Marshall & Marshall, 1985), although many more are believed to elude the attention of medical personnel (Doronzo, 1990).

During the normal course of development, many young children sustain blows to the head, the majority of which are of little or no concern (NHIF, 1985). Evidence suggests, however, that even minor concussions can produce actual damage to certain brain stem nuclei (Pang, 1985). In 1981, Rimel and her associates furnished clinical evidence that a mild concussion causing a brief loss of consciousness (less than 20 minutes) could produce both physiological and behavioral consequences. Memory, attention, and judgment showed disturbances as long as 3 months post injury. Gennarelli (1982) determined from his experimental study of acceleration-induced injuries that losses of consciousness (less than 2 minutes) produced momentary blood pressure and heart rate changes, an absence of corneal reflexes, and pronounced degenerative changes in the axons of reticular and vestibular nuclei and in dorsal regions of the medulla.

Although the term *concussion* has long been reserved for presumably pathology-free injuries that result in a transient loss of consciousness, support for this claim is strongly refuted (Alexander, 1984; Alves & Jane, 1985; Binder & Rattok, 1989; Boll, 1982, 1983; Levin, Benton, & Grossman, 1982). Jane and Rimel (1982), in their study of monkeys with mild concussion, confirmed the presence of degenerated axons in the brain stem reticular formation, colliculi, pons, and cerebral hemispheres. Pang's (1985) discussion of "minor concussive trauma," along with that of Alves and Jane (1985), strengthens the contemporary claim that mildly injured patients may be subject to permanent organic brain damage. Pang makes the point that minor injury is physiologically, as well as psychosocially, much more disabling than previously believed. There is considerable evidence to suggest that the effects of mild head injury are cumulative (Binder & Rattok, 1989). With each successive injury, the potential for permanent brain damage increases while the rate of recovery progressively decreases.

Mild head injuries may inhibit a child's ability to recall the moment of impact and the events that immediately follow (anterograde memory). The ability to recall the events that preceded the injury, however, remains intact (retrograde memory). Typically, those who sustain mild injury are conscious by the time they arrive at the emergency room and their neurological findings are normal (Friedman, 1983). Neurological findings are often superficially assessed following mild injuries so their absence does not necessarily confirm an absence of pathology (Boll, 1982). Contrast enhanced CT scans, if and when performed, frequently miss the minor lesions which accompany mild head injuries (Bakay & Glasauer, 1980; Baxter et al., 1985). An alteration of consciousness, no matter how brief, is indicative of brain injury (Jennett, 1979; Jennett & Teasdale, 1981) even though neurological findings may fail to detect physiological evidence (Alves & Jane, 1985; Boll, 1983; Doronzo, 1990).

Mild injuries can produce severe headaches, restlessness, disorientation, lethargy, irritability, withdrawal, apathy, and a reduced tolerance for stress (Boll, 1982, 1983). Such behavioral manifestations can set up a circle of negative reactions in the form of avoidance and rejection on the part of teachers, peers, and family. Once begun, this negative cycle may well continue beyond the life of the symptoms themsleves. Even so-called minor injuries can produce significant cognitive changes, such as impairment in attention, memory, and information processing, as well as changes in personality (Alves & Jane, 1985; Boll, 1982; Rimel et al., 1981). In a follow-up study by Klonoff et al. (1977), a significant proportion of mildly injured preschool and school-aged youngsters continued to show neurobehavioral deficits at 1 and 4 years post injury. Twenty-six percent failed a grade or were placed for the first time in remedial or "slow learner" classrooms subsequent to the injury.

A THI child may appear to be normal and fully recovered, yet continue to experience insidious behavioral, cognitive, emotional, and personality problems. Boll (1983) contends that IQ changes brought about by mild head injuries tend to be modest and remit relatively quickly, that is, within a few weeks to several months. Language deficits, memory, and attention difficulties may persist for 6 months or more. Information processing difficulties following mild injuries, on the other hand, exceed the limits of all other sequelae and may continue for several years.

Clearly, educational teams must recognize that mild injuries can produce consequences over which the child or adolescent has little or no control. Moreover, these consequences need to be viewed as symptoms worthy of individualized attention, prescribed methods of treatment, and, in some cases, related services (Boll, 1982;

Doronzo, 1990; Klonoff et al., 1977; Levin & Eisenberg, 1979; NHIF, 1985). It is not uncommon for school failure, behavioral maladjustment, and family disruption to escalate when educational systems underrate the significance of mild head injury in children and adolescents (Boll, 1982; Ylvisaker, 1985).

Moderate Head Injury

Head injuries that result in a loss of consciousness or PTA of 1–24 hours (GCS 9–12) are moderate. Once consciousness is regained, the moderately injured are generally able to follow simple commands, but remain lethargic (Friedman, 1983).

Rimel and her associates (1982) found that moderate injuries can cause persistent headaches, memory problems, and impairment in activities of daily living for as long as 3 months post injury. Of 199 moderately injured patients studied (aged 9 months to 60+ years) only 7% were found to be asymptomatic at 3 months. Sixty-nine percent had not resumed previous employment. Unemployment at 3 months post injury was twice that of mildly injured patients. Thirty-eight percent had made a "good" recovery although continued to experience headaches, memory problems, and difficulties in routine acts of daily living. Recipients of moderate head injury, compared to those whose injuries were mild, tended to be members of a lower socioeconomic class and showed a higher incidence of alcohol abuse and previous trauma. This trend was repeated in a comparison of moderately to severely injured patients. Severely injured patients tended to be even less affluent on the whole, were less educated, and had a history of even greater alcohol abuse and previous injury. Studies suggest a relationship between the occurrence of head injury and premorbid psychological disorders, alcohol use, learning disabilities, conduct disorders, and familial discord. Furthermore, children who sustain one head injury are at increased risk for sustaining another (Frankowski, 1986; Naugle, 1990).

Not only are moderate injuries more severe than mild injuries as measured by the GCS, but, as was found in Rimel's study, the incidence of hematomas and edema and the need for intracranial surgery is also greater. Neuropsychological assessment was conducted on 32 of Rimel's patients (aged 15 to 65) by means of the *Halstead-Reitan Neuropsychological Test Battery* (also known as the *Halstead-Reitan Battery*), *Wechsler Adult Intelligence Scale, Wide Range*

Achievement Test, and *Wechsler Memory Scale.* The results, although not necessarily representative of the entire patient population due to small sample size, revealed significant impairment on all measures of the Halstead-Reitan Battery, including tests of higher cognitive functioning, new problem-solving skills, memory, focused attention, and concentration. In simple terms, it may be concluded from these data that individuals who sustain a moderate injury are much worse off than those with mild injuries, yet tend to fare better than those who sustain severe injuries.

Severe Head Injury

Injuries resulting in a loss of consciousness or PTA of more than 24 hours (GCS 3-8) are considered severe (Frankowski et al., 1985). Patients with severe injuries are likely to require immediate, intricate, and systematic medical treatment such as mechanical ventilation, intravenous therapy, and/or neurosurgery (Bakay & Glasauer, 1980; North, 1984).

School-aged persons with severe injuries frequently experience persistent intellectual impairment and personality change, and are at increased risk for developing psychiatric disorder (Rutter, 1981). Scholastic achievement is often significantly affected. Ewing-Cobbs, Fletcher, and Levin (1985) identified specific deficits in confrontation naming, object description, verbal fluency, and writing to dictation. Children were more impaired than adolescents on measures of written language. Levin and Eisenberg (1979) consider memory impairment the most common cognitive deficit following closed head injury. Behavioral abnormalities, sensory and motor impairment, disturbances in attention and planning are also common (Alexander, 1984; Brink et al., 1980; Jaffe, Mastrilli, Molitor, & Valko, 1985).

Heiskanen and Kaste (1974) estimate that only 50% of those whose coma lasts more than two weeks can be expected to learn at a normal rate, or do even moderately well. A 4- to 10-year follow-up study of 36 youngsters with severe head injury revealed that, of the 34 who were school-aged, eight (24%) were unable to attend regular school programs following the injury and were permanently disabled (see Table 5). Nine (26%) returned to school but performed well below their preaccident level. Seven of these were considered to be doing adequate work in junior high school, but could not pass

TABLE 5

LENGTH OF COMA, SCHOOL PERFORMANCE, AND NEUROLOGICAL DEFICIT AFTER SEVERE BRAIN INJURY

Length of coma (days)	No. of cases	Educationally subnormal	Elementary school		High school		Hemiparesis	Epilepsy
			Poor progress	Fair success	Poor progress	Fair success		
1–2	4	—	—	1	2	—	1	1
3–7	14	2	3	6	—	2	3	—
8–14	9	1	1	6	—	1	3	3
15–30	6	2	2	1	1	—	2	—
30+	3	3	—	—	—	—	3	1
Totals	36	8	6	14	3	3	12	5

Note. "Late Prognosis of Severe Brain Injury in Children" by O. Heiskanen and M. Kaste, 1974, *Developmental Medicine and Child Neurology, 16,* p. 12. Copyright 1974 by MacKeith Press. Reprinted by permission.

TABLE 6

CHANGE IN INTELLECTUAL ABILITIES FOLLOWING SEVERE HEAD INJURY

Case No.	Age at injury	Days Coma	Days PTA	Years since injury	Estimated intelligence Before	Estimated intelligence After	Follow-up performance
1	5	35	56	10	Average (father a physician)	IQ 90. Rote memory poor. Wide scatter	Slow section ninth grade. Poor at complex tasks. [Poor motivation]
2	5	21	25+	8	[High] average	Average. Wide scatter. Poor rote memory	Reading difficulties. Increasing difficulty with complex tasks. [Left hemiplegia]
3	5	28	28+	13	Average	Low average. No intelligible speech. Wide scatter	Athetoid quadriplegic. Sixth-grade work; improving. [Types with head stick]
4	6	28	53	4	Average	IQ 65–70. Wide scatter. Poor rote memory	Special class, second-grade level. [Dysarthria. Right hemiparesis]
5	7	35	56	2	High average. Advanced group in class	Low average (IQ 80–89). Concrete, perseverative	Third grade. Reads well. Very distractible. Improving. [Now prefers left hand]
6	7	30	30+	3	Average	Low average. Wide scatter. Poor rote memory	Third grade. Poor reader. Poor comprehension. [Clumsy]

(continued)

TABLE 6
(CONTINUED)

Case No.	Age at injury	Days Coma	Days PTA	Years since injury	Estimated intelligence Before	Estimated intelligence After	Follow-up performance
7	11	47	65+	11	Average. Fifth grade	Low average. Scatter. Poor rote memory. Reads poorly	Finished high school. Responsible semi-skilled job. [Right hemiparesis]
8	14	42	60	1	Low average. Repeated fourth grade	IQ 70–80. Concrete. Poor rote memory	Slow eighth grade. Poor reader. Slow improvement. [Speech and language deficits]
9	16	35	56	3	IQ 115. Class leader	IQ 80. Very wide scatter. Perseverative	Parkinsonism. Expelled two schools. Psychiatric care in third school. [Violent]
10	18	7	64+	2	IQ 95–100. Behavior problems	IQ 70–80. Poor comprehension	Special high school. Improving. Unrealistic future goals. [Frustrated]

Note. Post traumatic amnesia includes coma.
Note. From "Some Effects of Severe Head Injury" by F. Richardson, 1963, *Developmental Medicine and Child Neurology, 5,* p. 476. Copyright 1963 by MacKeith Press. Reprinted by permission with adaptations.

a high school readiness exam. For the remaining 17 (50%), school performance was "fairly normal." Hemiparesis persisted in 12 patients. Five patients developed late epilepsy. Examination of the data reveals that subnormal educational progress was guaranteed for those whose comas extended beyond 30 days. Stover and Zeiger (1976) suspect that full recovery to preinjury status is unlikely following comas of 7 days or more. Even comas lasting for 3 or 4 days can induce a severe deterioration in intellectual capacity (Heiskanen & Kaste, 1974).

Richardson (1963) examined 10 school-aged patients (5–18 years) with severe closed head injuries (PTA > 7 days) for intellectual and neurological sequelae. A 2-day follow-up study at 2 years incorporated data from patient, family, and teacher interviews; and medical, neurological, and psychological measures (see Table 6). The instruments used for psychological evaluation included the *Wechsler Intelligence Scale for Children, Peabody Picture Vocabulary Test,* and *Stanford-Binet Intelligence Scale.* Preaccident IQ's were estimated on the basis of school records, parent interview, developmental milestones, and, when available, previous measures of IQ. When interviewed, all parents noted marked changes in the personalities of their children. They specifically noted increased anxiety, irritability, excessive fatigue, lability, poor concentration, and impaired memory. IQs at follow-up fell within the borderline to low-average limits, suggesting a decrement of 10 to 30 points from preinjury status. Deterioration in school performance of varying degrees was documented for all 10 students. Richardson also noted that the data in no way adequately reflected the devastating psychological effects of the injury upon these children and their families.

Mahoney and associates (1983) conducted a study of 46 severely head-injured patients aged 1–15 years. Twelve (26%) died within 10 days (mean = 2.5 days). Of the 12, 4 were pronounced dead on arrival, 4 died of internal injuries, and 4 died of secondary complications. The average length of PTA was greater than 15 days. Follow-up was conducted between 9 months and 4 years post injury (see Table 7 for outcomes).

The process of recovery from a severe head injury continues over a long period of time with some studies reporting notable improvements at 5 and 6 years post injury (Beaumont, 1983; Klonoff et al.,

TABLE 7

OUTCOMES OF 46 CHILDREN WITH SEVERE HEAD INJURY

# of Children (%)	Outcome of Follow-up
12 (26%)	Died of severe head trauma
3 (7%)	Severely handicapped; subnormal IQ; severe motor disability or persistent vegetative state
3 (7%)	Moderate motor handicap requiring aid in ambulation; borderline to normal IQ
18 (39%)	Mild learning or behavioral problems due to cerebral dysfunction; no neurologic deficit; borderline to normal IQ
10 (21%)	Returned to original school placement without behavioral or neurologic complaint

1977; Luria, 1963). Nevertheless, it is generally accepted that the most important period of recovery in children is the first 12 to 18 months, although significant improvements are possible during the second and third years (Beaumont, 1983; Rutter et al., 1983). Barth and Macciocchi (1985) estimate that approximately 85% of all cognitive/behavioral recovery following head trauma takes place within the first 18 months beyond coma. Alexander (1984) states that the time course of recovery following severe head injury is slow and generally includes one rapid period of improvement after the confusional state clears. Whether a plateau of recovery is ever reached following severe head injury is questionable. Such functions as memory, attention, and the ability to plan goals may never fully recover.

4

NEUROANATOMY AND BRAIN FUNCTION

An appreciation of the physiological and neuropsychological correlates of traumatic brain injury, the dynamic nature of brain functioning, and the recovery process is best obtained from a functional understanding of neuropsychology and neuroanatomy. This chapter offers a cursory sketch of the brain's structural composition, the arrangement of the central nervous system, functional localization theory, and neurodevelopmental principles. It has been included to provide the reader with a convenient review of basic neuropsychological and neuroanatomical concepts relevant to the study of traumatic head injury. Because of its superficial and selective nature, this chapter should not be used to take the place of a more detailed and comprehensive study such as would be available from the standard references of Beaumont (1983), Walsh (1978), Lezak (1983), Liebman (1986), or Kolb and Whishaw (1980, 1989).

The brain's chief product is behavior. Brain activity underlying any organized behavior is complex and involves countless neural interactions (Lezak, 1983). For example, the complex act of reading this page involves an extensive network of neurons (Luria, 1966). Discrete neurological activities such as the movement of a finger, however, can be disrupted by specific lesions to a particular area of the brain (Lezak, 1983). The disruption of complex behavior by brain lesions also occurs with enough regularity to make it possible to anticipate certain dysfunctions (e.g., the ability to copy a design) when the site of lesion is known (Luria, 1970a) and vice versa (Levin et al., 1985).

Functional localization or the localization of dysfunction implies a one-to-one correspondence between behavior and neuroanatomical site (Kolb & Whishaw, 1980; Luria, 1963). Such was the premise originally espoused by early localization theorists who were among the first to suggest that for every behavior or function, there exists a specific and corresponding neuroanatomical site responsible for its execution (Broca, 1865). Opponents of localization theory hypothesized brain functioning to be an *equipotential* process (Head, 1926; Lashley, 1937). Equipotential theorists contended that "functional areas" work together as a single integrated unit with shared responsibilities (Kolb & Whishaw, 1980). Hence, the effects of brain lesions would depend not upon their location, but upon their extent (Beaumont, 1983). *Functional system theory* (Geschwind, 1974b; Luria, 1970a) is the position accepted by most contemporary neuropsychologists. Its proponents recognize that certain functions are localized (e.g., primary sensory and motor functions) and that some operate on an equipotential basis (Beaumont, 1983). Higher level functions such as rational and abstract thinking are built up from a number of more basic component skills. While these component skills may be relatively localized, the variety of ways in which they are linked to comprise higher intellectual functions precludes point-to-point localization (Golden, 1981b; Tarter & Edwards, 1986). A functional system may be thought of as a chain with each link of the chain representing a particular area of the brain. If any segment of the functional system is broken, the behavior represented by the chain is disrupted (Golden, 1981b).

Brain Structure and Composition

The brain, which is 75% water, takes up approximately 80% of the space within the skull. The remaining 20% is occupied by cerebrospinal fluid (CSF), blood, cerebral arteries and veins (Jennett & Teasdale, 1981). Brain tissue is the most delicate of all body tissues (Liebman, 1986). Three membranes (meninges) protect the brain (see Figure 2). The closest meninge to the brain is the *pia mater.* The subarachnoid space which separates the pia mater from the second meninge, the *arachnoid,* is filled with CSF. Cerebrospinal fluid is a clear, colorless solution of sodium chloride and other salts which cushions the brain against trauma and provides a pathway for

FIGURE 2

PROTECTIVE LAYERS OF THE BRAIN

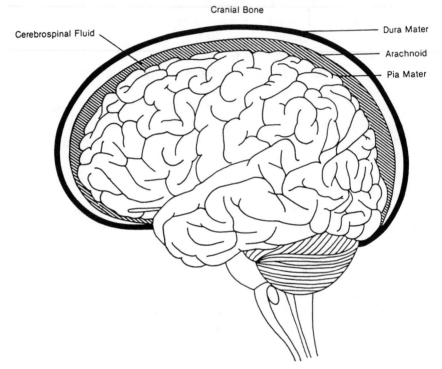

chemicals to reach the brain (Brookshire, 1978). CSF is continually produced by specialized tissues within each of four interconnected cavities called ventricles (Kolb & Whishaw, 1980; Lezak, 1983). The ventricles are numbered I to IV; the first and second ventricles are conventionally referred to as the lateral ventricles. Deterioration of brain substance may cause the ventricles to enlarge to fill the void (Beaumont, 1983). Thus, the size of ventricles can be an important early indicator of brain status. Enlarged ventricles are a common complication of closed head injury (Levin et al., 1981). The *dura mater* serves as the outer most meninge of the brain and lining for the inner surface of the cranial cavity.

At any given time, the brain contains approximately 20% of the body's total blood supply and consumes about 25% of the total oxygen supply required for the body (Brookshire, 1978). Because the brain has no metabolic or oxygen reserves, it is completely dependent upon blood for its oxygen and metabolic elements. If the blood supply to the brain is interrupted for more than 10 seconds, consciousness is lost. Permanent tissue damage occurs if the brain's blood supply is interrupted for more than 3 minutes (Brookshire, 1978; Jennett & Teasdale, 1981).

The brain itself is an intricately patterned collection of nerve cell bodies (neurons); fibers (axons and dendrites) that extend from nerve cell bodies and act as transmission organs; and support cells or glia (Lezak, 1983; Rourke et al., 1983) (see Figure 3). *Dendrites* collect and carry information toward the cell body; *axons* carry information away from the cell body (Brookshire, 1978). *Synapses* are the junctions between the end feet of a neuron and another cell. Synapses contain packages of chemical substances (neurotransmitters) that when released influence the activity of other cells. When a neuron fires, neurotransmitters are released which bind to receptor membranes to form a connection with another cell. The neurotransmitters are then quickly washed away by extracellular fluid and are either destroyed or taken back for reuse (Kolb & Whishaw, 1980).

FIGURE 3

TWO NEURONS IN SYNAPTIC CONTACT

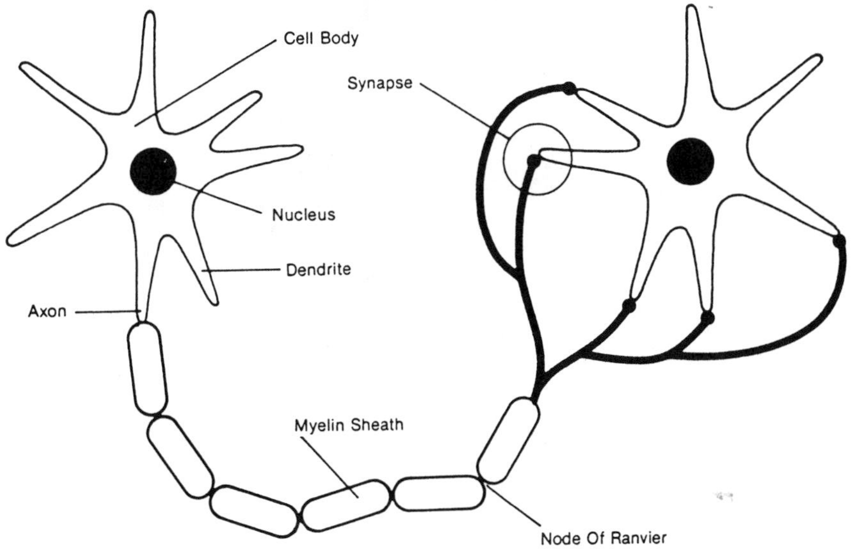

43

Anatomy of the Central Nervous System

The central nervous system can be divided into six component parts (Rourke et al., 1983).

1. The *spinal cord* is a long cylindrical structure made up of 31 pairs of spinal nerves which are encased in the vertebrae of the spine. The cord receives information from the skin and muscles in localized areas of the body and relays motor commands for movement.

2. The *brain stem* which extends upward from the spinal cord is composed of three regions, the medulla, pons, and midbrain (see Figure 4). The reticular formation (also known as the reticular activating system, RAS) is a complex network of cell bodies and fibers which begins at the upper end of the spinal cord and runs through the brain stem. This network mediates

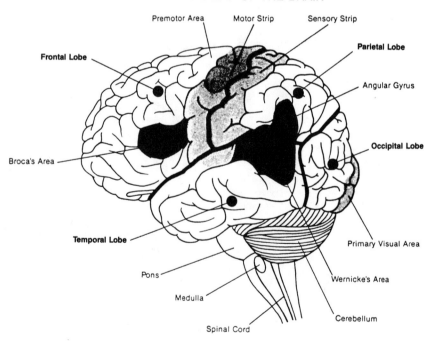

FIGURE 4

ORGANIZATIONAL MAP OF THE BRAIN

postural reflexes and is associated with arousal. Lesions involving the reticular formation typically result in global disorders of consciousness.

3. The *cerebellum* overlaps the pons and medulla to connect with the brain stem. This structure is primarily involved with the maintenance of equilibrium and muscle tone, and movement modulation.

4. The *basal ganglia* are composed of the putamen, caudate, and globus pallidus and are involved in modulating and modifying motor movements. Damage to basal ganglia results in involuntary motor movements, and changes in posture, or disturbances in muscle tone (Kolb & Whishaw, 1980).

5. The *diencephalon* includes the thalamus, hypothalamus, subthalamus, and epithalamus. These structures are responsible for transmitting information regarding sensation and movement. The hypothalamus, in particular, exercises control over such functions as body temperature, water metabolism, hormonal secretions, blood pressure, hunger, and sleep (Liebman, 1986). It also maintains a close association with the limbic system and plays a role in emotional reactions.

6. The *cortex* caps the entire system and is divided into two halves or hemispheres. Each hemisphere is divided into four regions or lobes, namely, the frontal, parietal, temporal, and occipital lobes. The white matter of the cerebral hemispheres consists of densely packed conduction fibers that transmit neural impulses between cortical points within a hemisphere (association fibers), between hemispheres (commissural fibers), or between the cortex and lower levels (projection fibers). Projection fibers can be divided into afferent (sensory) and efferent (motor) fibers. Afferent fibers receive sensory information and relay it toward the brain. Efferent fibers arise from the motor and premotor areas of the cortex and travel downward through the brain stem and spinal cord before they are distributed to the various body parts and areas they serve.

The corpus callosum is the great band of commissural fibers which connects the two hemispheres and allows for rapid and effective interhemisphere communication (Lezak, 1983). With the exception of the visual and auditory systems, the primary centers of each hemisphere mediate the activities of the contralateral (opposite) side of the body. Thus, an injury affecting the left motor strip will result in a right-sided weakness or paralysis.

Visual sensations are transmitted from the retina to the occipital lobe. Each eye has two visual fields, namely, a temporal and nasal field, which are further divided into upper and lower sections. Each eye can be conceived as having four quadrants (see Figure 5). A visual pathway consists of an optic nerve, its fibers which travel through or along the sides of the optic chiasm, and an optic tract. Each optic nerve contains fibers from only one retina. The optic chiasm contains fibers from the nasal sections of each retina. These fibers cross to the opposite side of the brain at the optic chiasm (Urdang & Swallow, 1983). The fibers from the temporal portion of each eye do not cross at the optic chiasm; rather, they travel along the same side of the brain en route to the occipital lobe. The optic tracts, optic chiasm, and occipital lobe each contain nerve fibers from both eyes. Simply stated, the visual system is organized according to a bilateral scheme. The left visual field of each eye is represented on the right occipital cortex, and the right visual fields are represented on the left occipital cortex (Beaumont, 1983; Brookshire, 1978; Liebman, 1986). If, for example, the right optic tract is damaged, partial vision will be lost in both eyes, namely, the left temporal and right nasal fields of vision.

The majority of nerve fibers transmitting auditory stimulation from each ear are projected to the primary auditory centers in the opposite hemisphere. The remaining fibers travel to the ipsilateral (same-sided) auditory cortex (Lezak, 1983). If the left auditory cortex is damaged, the patient will continue to hear from both ears using the intact right auditory cortex. Damage to the left or right auditory nerve, however, will cause total deafness in the corresponding ear (Liebman, 1986).

Dynamic Functional Localization

The late Alexander R. Luria, famed Russian neuropsychologist, has been recognized as a major force behind modern day neuropsychology (Luria, 1963, 1966, 1969, 1970a, b, 1973). His theory of cerebral organization was the impetus behind the posthumous

FIGURE 5

VISUAL FIELDS

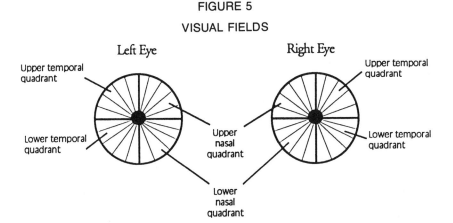

development of a standardized battery of neuropsychological tests, the *Luria-Nebraska Neuropsychological Battery* (Golden, Hammeke, & Purisch, 1980). Because of Luria's extensive work with brain-damaged patients and his understanding of brain pathology and function, his theories remain highly relevant to the study of THI and merit discussion. At the core of Luria's work was his theory of brain function (Golden, 1981b; Reynolds, 1981). He conceptualized the brain as being organized into three major units or "blocks": (1) the arousal unit, (2) the sensory input unit, and (3) the output/ planning unit. (See Table 8).

1. *Block one.* As illustrated, the first block is composed of the brain stem including the reticular formation, midbrain, pons, and medulla. Together these parts make up the reticular activating system (RAS). The first block is reponsible for regulating the energy level and tone of all portions of the cortex. It regulates consciousness and provides a stable basis for the organism to structure various functions and processes.

The reticular formation is responsible for filtering sensory input, arousal, and activation within the cortex. Injuries to the first block of the brain or any interruption of impulses between the first block and the cortex results in an alteration or loss of consciousness.

2. *Block two.* Most of the cognitive information processing of the brain takes place within the second block. The temporal lobes are responsible for the reception, analysis, and encoding of auditory stimuli; the occipital lobes receive, analyze, and encode visual stimuli;

TABLE 8

DYNAMIC FUNCTIONAL LOCALIZATION: LURIA'S THEORY
OF BRAIN FUNCTION

Blocks	Composition	Function
(1) "Arousal Unit"	BRAINSTEM: RETICULAR FORMATION; MIDBRAIN; PONS; MEDULLA	—arousal —consciousness —activation of cortical functions
(2) "Sensory Input Unit"	TEMPORAL, OCCIPITAL, PARIETAL LOBES "association cortex"	—sorting and recording —sequential organization and coding —simultaneous processing, integration
	specific ← ↑↓ → integrated A. Primary Zone—receives, sorts, records information B. Secondary Zone—organizes, codes information C. Tertiary Zone—merges, synthesizes, forms basis of complex behavior	
(3) "Output/ Planning Unit"	FRONTAL LOBES "executor"	—formulation of intentions and programs of behavior —higher order processing —locus of intelligence
	specific ← ↑↓ → integrated A. Primary Zone (motor output): "motor strip," "motor cortex"— sends motor commands to muscles B. Secondary Zone (premotor area) —organizes the sequences of motor acts C. Tertiary Zone (prefrontal lobes)— maturity, decision making, planning, attention, delay of gratification	

the parietal lobes receive, analyze, and encode kinesthetic and tactile information. Each lobe is organized into three hierarchical areas, namely, the primary, secondary, and tertiary zones. Of all the areas of the cortex, the primary zones are the closest to being "hard wired." In other words, input is localized within the primary zone in direct one-to-one correspondence with the end-organ sense receptors — the eyes, ears, and skin. The primary zones of each lobe within the second block are capable of sorting and recording incoming sensory information. The secondary zones sequentially organize and code information passed on by the primary zone. For example, the secondary area of the occipital lobes analyzes stimuli for color, form, and shape and differentiates essential from nonessential visual stimuli. The three tertiary zones of block two are in close proximity. At their juncture within the left hemisphere (Wernicke's area and the angular gyrus), multiple sources of input are fused and analyzed simultaneously. This is the area believed responsible for cross-modality processing (Das, Kirby, & Jarman, 1979). Reading, arithmetic, writing, grammar, and logical analysis, among other skills, are mediated by the tertiary zones of the second block (Golden, 1981b).

Damage to the second block of the brain can lead to the loss or impairment of any one of the aforementioned functions. For example, damage to the primary zone of the occipital lobe may result in a visual disturbance. Cortical blindness (or deafness) occurs when both primary zones of the occipital (or temporal) lobes are completely destroyed. Damage to the tertiary zones may disrupt the ability to integrate across two or three sensory systems, resulting in such symptoms as anomia (word-finding difficulties), dyslexia (severe reading impairment), dysgraphia (writing disturbances), or dyspraxia (severe problems in motor coordination) (Beaumont, 1983; Golden, 1981b).

3. *Block three.* The third block of the brain, comprising the frontal lobes, is involved with higher order processing such as the organization, conscious implementation, and formation of intentions and programs of behavior (Luria, 1970a). It, too, is subdivided into primary, secondary, and tertiary zones. The frontal lobes, which have no responsibility for simple sensory or motor functions (Luria, 1970a), are closely associated with the reticular formation and are also involved with the activation and regulation of the remainder of the cortex. The frontal lobes are considered the "executive branch" and anatomical locus of intelligence.

The primary zone of the frontal lobe is referred to as the motor output area of the brain (also called "motor cortex" and "motor strip"). Commands are sent from this area to the specific muscles needed to perform motor acts, including speech functions. Damage to the motor cortex can result in deficits of fine motor control and strength of limbs, or a reduction in speech functions (Beaumont, 1983). The secondary (premotor) area is responsible for organizing the sequence of these motor acts. The primary and secondary zones of the output/planning unit interact cooperatively to signal and organize movement. Injuries to the motor area of the brain can produce hemiplegia (paralysis to one side of the body), or speech disorders such as dysfluency (e.g., stuttering).

The tertiary area of the third block of the brain is commonly referred to as the prefrontal lobes. It is responsible for long-range planning (decision making), evaluation, impulse control, selective attention, creativity, and maturity (Golden, 1981b). As the prefrontal lobes begin to develop (around puberty) they assume dominance over the arousal unit of the brain (reticular system). At this point, the responsibility for regulating attention and arousal, once assumed by the first block, is relinquished to the prefrontal lobes (Reynolds, 1981).

Simply put, Luria theorized that the cortex works in the following way: Sensory input which enters the primary zones is elaborated and analyzed by the respective secondary zones and integrated in the tertiary zones. For an action to be executed, information from the occipital, temporal, and parietal tertiary zones is sent to the tertiary zone of the output/planning unit (block three), then to its secondary zone and finally to the primary zone (motor strip) where the commands for behavior are sent to specific muscles.

Using Luria's concept of cortical functioning, brain lesions can be conceived as having three distinct effects upon behavior: (a) the loss of function, (b) the release of function, or (c) the disorganization of function (Kolb & Whishaw, 1980). The most obvious effect of brain damage is the loss of function. As a general rule, the larger the lesion the greater the loss (Kolb & Whishaw, 1980), although it does not necessarily follow that small lesions produce relatively minor losses. Damage to certain critical areas of the brain can produce dramatic consequences regardless of relative size (e.g., damage to speech or language centers) (Barth & Boll, 1981). A release of function occurs when a new behavior appears or when the frequency of a behavior is increased (e.g., tremors, perseverative behaviors, disinhibition). The disorganization of function is exemplified by the person who has maintained the ability to execute the individual steps of a complex behavior, but who is unable to sequence the behavior in an organized and practical way.

Stages of Neurodevelopment

Neurodevelopmental theory affords professionals a basis by which to comprehend more fully the significance of age-at-injury upon outcome. The schematic model of cognitive neurodevelopment (see Figure 6) shows the progressive nature of hemispheric specialization for complex cognitive functions. Both hemispheres tend to share responsibility for simple cognitive functions during the first five years. Between the ages of 5 and 8 years, the left and right hemispheres of most individuals begin to specialize in certain verbal and nonverbal functions, respectively. This does not indicate,

FIGURE 6

PROGRESSIVE SPECIALIZATION OF COMPLEX
FUNCTIONS BY LEFT AND RIGHT HEMISPHERES

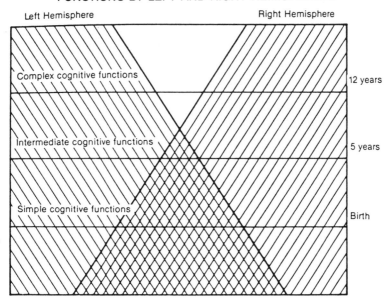

however, that the hemispheres develop functional independence with maturity. Rather, both begin to take on the respective responsibilities for which they were innately assigned (Kolb & Whishaw, 1980). They continue to work cooperatively on a number of functions and maintain a synergistic relationship. Both hemispheres share responsibility for most intellectual functions yet are capable of making separate cognitive contributions. Table 9 lists the principal functions of the left and right hemispheres. The list was derived from observations of patients with lateralized brain damage, split brain studies, and experimental investigations of hemispheric preferences (Cummings, 1985).

Golden (1981b) identifies five distinct stages of neurodevelopment during which qualitative changes in cognitive abilities occur. Embedded in this developmental framework is the premise that a child must achieve a certain stage of physiological development and be given the environmental opportunity for such development to be considered capable of performing certain cognitive operations. The five major stages of neurodevelopment follow.

Stage 1. (Development of the arousal unit). The reticular system is generally operative by birth and fully operational within 12 months of conception.

Stage 2. (Development of the primary motor and sensory areas). The neurological development of the four primary (motor and

TABLE 9

FUNCTIONS ATTRIBUTABLE TO EACH CEREBRAL HEMISPHERE

	Left	**Right**
Language	Speaking aloud	Auditory comprehension
	Auditory comprehension	Reading comprehension
	Naming	Prosodic expression
	Reading comprehension	Prosodic comprehension
	Reading aloud	
	Writing	
Constructions	Internal detail	External configurations
Calculations	Arithmetic processing	Spatial arrangement
Memory	Verbal	Visuospatial
Miscellaneous	Skilled movements	Facial recognition

sensory) areas of the brain is generally complete within 12 months of conception.

Stage 3. (Development of the secondary motor and sensory areas). This stage begins at conception and continues through age 5 years. It is during this level that the first important differentiation of the brain into verbal and nonverbal hemispheres occurs. Capacity for coordinated movement, visual and auditory recognition, sensory discrimination, and the association of objects with words develops (Lehr, 1990a). By 2 years of age, 93% of the population develops a left hemisphere that is specialized for the mediation of language-related functions (Milner, 1975). In general, serious damage to the left hemisphere prior to age 2 will result in a transfer of responsibility for verbal skills to the right hemisphere. During the first 5 years of life, integrative (cross-modality) processing is not possible because the tertiary zones have not yet developed.

Stage 4. (Development of the tertiary areas of the second block). The tertiary areas of the temporal, occipital, and parietal lobes become psychologically active between 5 and 8 years of age. The tertiary areas accommodate the linkage of auditory, visual, and tactile perceptions and are responsible for the integration of information required for reading, arithmetic, written language, reasoning by analogy, and categorizing (Lehr, 1990a). In effect, damage to the tertiary areas can seriously inhibit academic learning by compromising the ability to integrate simultaneously two or more sensory modalities (Luria, 1966).

Stage 5. (Development of the output/planning unit or prefrontal lobes). During this final stage, the maturation and elaboration of the frontal lobes occurs. As this is the last cortical area to develop (beginning at about age 12 and continuing through age 24), its susceptibility to damage is highly pronounced. Preadolescent damage to the frontal lobes may not surface until the frontal lobes become operational. Consequently, the effects of earlier occurring injuries often surface at a later stage of development and can interfere with the adolescent's formulation of intentions, long-range planning, impulse control, cognitive flexibility, decision making, and social maturity.

Piaget's stages of cognitive development (1969) elucidate the transformation of concrete to formal thinking and provide a functional parallel to neurodevelopmental maturation. According to

Piaget, primitive interactions with the environment occur at a sensory and motor level during the *sensorimotor* stage (0–2 years). During the *preoperational* stage (2–7 years), properties such as height, weight, length, and color are processed on a simplistic and unidimensional plane. Logical deductions and operations become possible during the *concrete operational* stage (7–11 years); concepts are no longer perceived as having unitary sensory features alone, and simple generalizations and simultaneous conceptualizations are possible. During the *formal operations* stage (11–15 years), the ability to recognize and consider complex relationships and make comprehensive judgments emerges. Multiple concepts can be processed simultaneously (Kohen-Raz, 1977; Strang, 1983).

5

OUTCOME AND RECOVERY

Reference to outcome in this chapter (and elsewhere in the text) implies both *mortality* (death, rate of death) and *morbidity* (an abnormal condition of quality) (Urdang & Swallow, 1983). Recovery refers to the transitory phase and conditions that take place between the insult and the point at which no symptoms of the injury remain.

Categories of Outcome

The need for a reliable method of categorizing outcomes following traumatic head injury prompted Jennett and Bond (1975) to devise the *Glasgow Outcome Scale* (GOS). The GOS makes it possible to make discrete comparisons between surviving individuals and between groups of survivors (Eisenberg, 1985). The medical profession makes use of GOS terms to distinguish possible outcomes. The GOS stratifies outcome into four categories on the basis of overall social capability or dependence. Although individual categorizations are determined subjectively, the differences between levels are sufficiently broad, and, as such, reduce the likelihood of inter-rater disagreement (Jennett & Teasdale, 1981). The four survival categories of the GOS are:

1. *Vegetative State.* A "vegetative state" implies an absence of cerebral cortical function (Jennett & Bond, 1975). Diffuse cerebral hypoxia or severe shearing lesions in the white matter are generally responsible for producing a persistent vegetative state (Jennett &

Teasdale, 1981). Patients in this state may be able to open their eyes and show a grasp reflex, but are unable to speak or respond in any meaningful way. Higashi et al. (1977) further clarified the vegetative state as indicative of urinary and fecal incontinence, a complete loss of self-supportability, and the absence of expressive intent and emotional expression. A persistent vegetative state does not imply, however, that further improvement is impossible; in fact, many patients pass through and beyond this state during the course of their recovery (Levin, Benton, & Grossman, 1982).

2. *Severe Disability.* This condition implies severe functional disability. Individuals who fall into this category are dependent on some other person for daily support because of mental and/or physical disability (Jennett & Bond, 1975; Jennett & Teasdale, 1981). These individuals are often institutionalized or cared for at home. The worst affected often display marked paralysis, dysarthria and dysphasia, and severely restricted mental ability. Some may be capable of limited communication, ambulation, and self-care but invariably require close vigilance and supervision (Jennett & Teasdale, 1981; Levin, Benton, & Grossman, 1982).

3. *Moderate Disability.* These individuals are considered "independent" but disabled. They are able to travel by public transport and some are capable of work (usually, but not necessarily, within a sheltered environment). Moderately disabled persons show persistent motor and neuropsychological deficits and major personality changes. Persons who are moderately disabled may have been severely disabled during their first year of recovery (Levin, Benton, & Grossman, 1982; Jennett & Bond, 1975).

4. *Good Recovery.* This category does not necessarily imply the restoration of all normal functions as considerable neuropsychological impairment frequently persists. Mild impairment on some psychological tests and mild behavioral disturbances may remain. The IQs of these individuals generally recover to within average limits. Approximately one-third to one-half of the survivors of severe closed head injury can achieve a good recovery (Levin, Benton, & Grossman, 1982).

Based upon a study of general recovery curves, Teasdale and Jennett (1976) recommend that assessment of outcome by means of the Glasgow Outcome Scale be conducted at six months post injury. Jennett, Teasdale, Braakman, Minderhoud, and Knill-Jones

(1976) determined that the improvements occurring beyond 6 months were rarely significant enough to warrant a change in category, although this does indeed occur (Levin, Benton, & Grossman, 1982). Approximately two-thirds of the patients they studied who had achieved either good or moderate recovery at 1 year following the injury, had earned such a status within 3 months, whereas 90% had earned their one-year status within 6 months of the injury. These data should not be taken to mean that specific cognitive and behavioral improvements are rare or minimal beyond 6 months; the GOS was originally intended to serve as a *broad* measure of global change, and, as such, lacks a sensitivity for individual and specific improvements (Eisenberg, 1985; Rosenthal et al., 1983). Data from Jennett et al. (1976) show that 10% of the 150 patients studied who were severely or moderately disabled at 6 months did in fact move up to become moderate or good, respectively, within 1 year. Another 5% of 82 patients followed for more than 18 months showed additional improvement sufficient to upgrade outcome category after 1 year. In another similar study (see Table 10) of more than 500 survivors, recovery was rated at 3, 6, and 12 months by means of the GOS (Jennett & Teasdale, 1981). By the end of the first year, there were notably more "good" recoveries and progressively less "severely disabled" patients. This trend toward improvement was the result of at least two prominent factors: (a)

TABLE 10

SURVIVORS AFTER SEVERE HEAD INJURY

	Survivors at		
Outcome	3 months n = 534	6 months n = 515	12 months n = 376
Vegetative state	7%	5%	3%
Severe disability	29	19	16
Moderate disability	33	34	31
Good recovery	31	42	50
Moderate/Good	64	76	81

Note. From *Management of Head Injuries* (p. 309) by B. Jennett and G. Teasdale, 1981, Philadelphia: F. A. Davis Company. Copyright 1981 by F. A. Davis Co. Reprinted by permission.

genuine gains in social capability among groups, and (b) deaths within the severe and vegetative groups over the course of follow-up.

The outcomes of nearly 1,000 patients were studied by Jennett, Teasdale, Braakman, Minderhoud, Heiden, and Kurze (1979). Eighty-seven percent with original GCS scores of 11 or more made a moderate or good recovery. Sixty-eight percent with scores between 8 and 10, 34% percent with scores between 5 and 7, and 7% with scores of 3 or 4 made moderate or better recoveries.

Although the Glasgow Outcome Scale is particularly useful for stratifying outcomes and classifying recovery following THI, its suitableness for school-aged children is somewhat limited in the absence of school and developmentally related criteria (Levin, Ewing-Cobbs, & Benton, 1984). For this reason, outcome ratings for children should be supplemented by formal measures of cognitive functioning, behavior, motor function, achievement, social skills, personality, and neuropsychological functions (Boll, 1983; Lezak, 1983; Rosenthal et al., 1983).

Variables Related to Outcome

Numerous factors associated with the injury (degree and nature of primary damage, secondary or early neurological variables, causal agent, site of injury) and the individual (age, premorbid characteristics) interact to produce highly complex behavioral correlates (Lezak, 1983; Rourke, Bakker, Fisk, & Strang, 1983; Sattler, 1982). For this reason, it is difficult to make clear and meaningful distinctions about the predictive capability of any one variable in isolation. The fact that no two brains nor the injuries they sustain are alike further complicates prognoses. Moreover, the subsequent availability and quality of medical care, rehabilitative and educational programs, teachers and therapists, the residual resources of the child, and family attitudes have an immeasurable effect upon outcome and recovery (Evans, 1981; Rourke et al., 1983).

Variables associated with outcome following traumatic head injury will be discussed both in terms of morbidity and mortality. They are organized into two broad categories, namely, those directly related to the injury and those related to the individual.

Injury-Based Variables

Degree and Nature of Primary Damage. Even in the absence of pre-existing behavioral disturbances, individuals who sustain severe head injuries are at increased risk for developing behavioral complications (Klonoff & Low, 1974; Rutter et al., 1983). Cognitive impairment and a deterioriation in school performance are also common by-products of the most severe injuries (Chadwick, Rutter, Thompson, & Shaffer, 1981; Richardson, 1963). Severe diffuse brain injury has been found to be a primary determinant of cognitive residua in children and adolescents (Levin, Eisenberg, Wigg, & Kobayashi, 1982). Rutter et al. (1983) consider intellectual deficit a direct function of the severity of generalized brain damage. Levin, Benton, and Grossman (1982) determined that widespread damage creates long-term learning difficulties. Others have noted that diffuse brain damage results in a marked depression of Performance IQs, as well as severe motor and perceptual deficits (Rourke et al., 1983).

Death resulting from severe head injury usually occurs within 3 days of the injury (Eisenberg, 1985; Richardson, 1963). Patients who sustain severe head injuries (GCS < 9) have a 50-70% chance of survival given optimal medical therapy (Levin, Benton, & Grossman, 1982).

Neurological Determinants. Patients with lesions requiring surgical management have a higher mortality (55%) than those who do not (20%) according to Bowers and Marshall (1980). Ninety-five percent of those with elevated and nonreducible intracranial pressure (ICP) die, compared to a mortality of 19% for patients with normal ICP (Narayan et al., 1982). Early measures of somatosensory, auditory, auditory brain stem, and visual pathways (via multimodality evoked potentials [MEPs]) have been instrumental in predicting outcome at 1 year with 80% accuracy (Greenberg, Newlon, & Hyatt, 1981). Hence, MEPs are considered by some an impressively reliable predictor of outcome (Davis & Cunningham, 1984). Braakman, Gelpke, Habbema, Mass, and Minderhoud (1980), on the other hand, ranked the best predictors of outcome to be age, early pupillary responses, and the eye plus motor score from the GCS. Narayan et al. (1981) statistically determined from their studies that the five best predictors of outcome were: MEP, age, intracranial pressure data, Glasgow Coma Scale score, and pupillary response.

A relationship between early signs of ventricular enlargement and persistent cognitive impairment in adolescents who sustained closed head injury was found by Levin, Meyers, Grossman, and Sarwar (1981). Specifically, Levin and his colleagues found evidence of impaired learning abilities, IQs of less than 85, and word retention and memory difficulties at 5 months post injury in patients whose initial CT scans (taken within 30 days of the injury) revealed ventricular enlargement. Absent pupillary and oculocephalic responses (brain stem reflexes) and decerebrate rigidity (exaggerated extensor posture in all extremities caused by brain stem lesion) are almost always associated with impending death (70-90% mortality rate) (Davis & Davis, 1982; Levati, Farina, & Vecchi, 1982; Miller et al., 1981).

Causal Agent. Some discussion of the differences between brain injuries and sequelae following open (penetrating) injuries and those that result from acceleration/deceleration injuries to the head has been offered in chapter 2. Recovery from focal lesions due to skull penetration progresses more rapidly and reaches an earlier plateau than recovery following diffuse damage (Alexander, 1984). Epilepsy, however, is more likely to occur following focal injuries (Jennett, 1975a). Persistent sensory-motor deficits, by contrast, are more common among closed head injuries (Pang, 1985).

Motor vehicle accidents are the leading cause of head injury deaths in the United States. Gunshot wounds as a result of suicides and homicides are the second most common cause, with falls representing the third most prevalent death-producing mechanism. Other causes of head injury deaths are natural disasters, assaults, machinery, and air and railway transport accidents (Sosin, Sacks, & Smith, 1989) (see Figure 7).

Site of Injury. The brains of older adolescents and adults are more structurally refined than those of developing children. Consequently, the relationship that exists between site of damage and behavioral consequences is far more direct and reliable. As the brain matures, the pattern of cognitive and psychiatric sequelae and its association with specific lesions become increasingly more pronounced

FIGURE 7

CAUSES OF HEAD INJURY DEATHS IN THE UNITED STATES

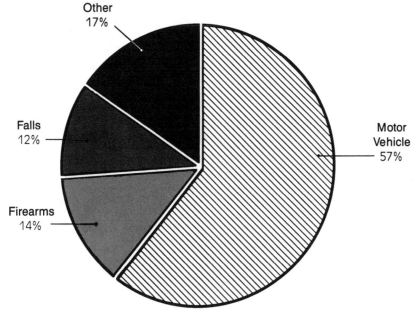

and predictable (Chadwick, Rutter, Thompson, & Shaffer, 1981; Lehr, 1990b; Lishman, 1968, 1978). Rutter (1981) concluded, however, that although cognitive deficits associated with lateralized (side-specific) brain lesions in children are broadly similar to those found in adolescents and adults, they tend to be less marked and less differentiated. In general, left hemisphere lesions tend to produce language and verbal deficits. Quantitatively, left-sided lesions depress both Verbal and Performance IQs (Kaufman et al., 1985; McFie, 1961, 1975; Rourke et al., 1983; Rutter, 1981). By contrast, right hemisphere lesions typically result in visual-spatial deficits and depress Performance IQs (Lezak, 1983). Unilateral damage to the motor area of the frontal lobe affects motor functions on the opposite side of the body, that is, on the side *contralateral* to the site of injury. The effects of lesion laterality are most pronounced immediately following the injury (Fitzhugh, Fitzhugh, & Reitan, 1962; Newcombe, 1969; Rutter et al., 1983).

Neuropathology and neuroimaging studies have determined that closed head injuries characteristically produce damage to the frontal

61

and temporal lobes (Levin, 1990). Given the functional responsibilities of the frontal and temporal lobes, it is not surprising that closed head injuries so often compromise problem-solving capabilities, higher order processing, initiative, memory, and new learning (Levin, 1990).

In a study of 670 patients with penetrating injuries, Lishman (1968) investigated the psychiatric effects of various lesion sites. Affective disorders, behavior abnormalities (e.g., disinhibition, lack of insight), and somatic complaints were more frequent following right-hemisphere lesions and frontal lobe damage. All forms of psychiatric sequelae were strongly associated with frontal lobe damage. Goldberger (1974) showed early evidence that monkeys recover to a greater extent from lesions to the premotor cortex (secondary) than from lesions to the motor cortex (primary) and subcortical areas of the motor system. In a study of human subjects, Rourke et al. (1983) concluded that degree of recovery is related to site of injury, with less recovery following the destruction of primary (earlier developing) zones as compared to secondary and tertiary projection areas. Rate and degree of recovery, therefore, correlate negatively with degree of specificity and the relative immaturity of the injured area.

Lower brain stem injuries produce severe physical disability, communication disorders, severe fatigability, and low arousal and drive. Lesions to the midbrain can cause emotional instability and affect the gestural expression of emotion. For example, midbrain lesions can produce an apparent mismatch between affect and outward expression (Eames, 1990).

Individual Differences

Age and Outcome. A comparison of recovery from traumatic head injury on the basis of age is complicated by the influences of neurodevelopmental stage, maturation, and hemispheric specialization (Rutter et al., 1983). The interaction of these processes, combined with the influences of the injury itself (Ewing-Cobbs et al., 1985) and individual characteristics such as premorbid IQ (Rutter et al., 1983) and acquired knowledge (Rourke et al., 1983), make it difficult to determine whether THI children as a group are "better" or "worse" off than THI adults. The greater cerebral plasticity (degree to which recovery of function is possible) of children and greater potential for an interhemispheric transfer of function in the immature brain makes a child's response to brain damage different from that of older, more committed brains (Rutter et al., 1983). An immature brain is less committed to specific functions. Consequently, undamaged areas may take on responsibility for a damaged part. For this reason, children will often show remarkable and rapid postinjury improvement. Recent findings indicate, however, that certain areas of the brain may be committed to certain functions as early as infancy. Furthermore, not all areas of the brain are capable of assuming all functions (Lehr, 1990a). As a form of recovery, the transfer of responsibility from damaged to undamaged part often leads to unusual neuronal connections, a diminution of the function originally assigned to the area that has assumed additional responsibility, and comparatively lesser quality cortical functioning overall (Lehr, 1990a).

Given that the skull of a young person is less rigid than that of an adult, greater cushioning effects are possible (Levin, Benton, & Grossman, 1982). By the same token, there is likely to be greater distortion in the young brain, hence, greater cause for shearing damage (Rutter et al., 1983). Children may be disproportionately affected by brain damage because the continued acquisition of skills is so dependent upon memory and memory impairment is the most common cognitive sequel of pediatric head injury (Levin et al., 1982; Levin & Eisenberg, 1979; Rutter, 1981).

Although some early childhood injuries may appear mild, their appearances are often deceptive; real evidence of deficit may surface later in life (Rourke, 1983). For example, a child may first experience problems associated with a prior injury when the functions subserved by the damaged tissue become crucial, that is, during a later stage of development. In other words, a child may grow into a deficit. Early lesions to the prefrontal lobes may not surface until the prefrontal area of the cortex becomes operational (between the ages of 12 and 24 years) (Golden, 1981b; Luria, 1963). Likewise, the manifestation of specific cognitive deficiencies, although present in young head-injured persons, may be masked by more obvious and pervasive attentional deficits (Rourke, 1983). Over time, these attentional deficits may subside only to be replaced by the neurobehavioral deficits they have masked. Rourke explains this process as similar to the secondary consequences produced by edema: as edema resolves, the generalized deficits it has produced subside, giving way to the original and underlying consequences of the primary focal damage. Rudel (1978) concludes that the effects of brain damage sustained during childhood may (a) appear initially then disappear, (b) appear initially and persist, or (c) surface during a more advanced stage of development. The pattern depends on such factors as the type of tissue destroyed, the functions involved, the environmental interaction experienced, and, most importantly, on the neurodevelopmental status and differentiation of the brain. The theories of Rourke and Rudel help explain why some children may begin to perform poorly after a period of apparent improvement.

There is considerable evidence to suggest that children exhibit more severe neurologic dysfunction than adolescents (Becker et al., 1977; Bruce, Schut, Bruno, Wood, & Sutton, 1978; Levin et al., 1984). This has been attributed to diffuse white matter damage and cerebral swelling (Bruce et al., 1978). With respect to language functions, however, Lenneberg (1967) determined that the potential for recovery from aphasia is better for children because language acquisition is dependent upon cerebral maturation. The prognosis for recovery from aphasia depreciates markedly with the onset of puberty, presumably due to the increased functional specialization of the left hemisphere for language (Shapiro, 1985) and the increasing committedness of the right hemisphere for nonlinguistic processes (Kinsbourne & Hiscock, 1981; Luria, 1970b; Rudel, 1978). As the cerebral hemispheres mature and become more specialized, the brain's capacity to transfer functional responsibility from one hemisphere to the other decreases (Hécaen, 1976; Woods, 1980). Levin and Eisenberg (1979) found in their follow-up study of 64 THI children and adolescents that young children showed an impressive recovery of oral language comprehension, whereas similar deficits persisted when injuries occurred during adolescence.

Levin, Eisenberg et al. (1982) found that severe head injuries cause greater intellectual impairment in children than they do in adolescents. It has also been determined that the restoration of memory after diffuse insult to the child's brain is slower and less complete than it is for adolescents (Gaidolfi & Vignolo, 1980).

Children under 10 years of age were shown to exhibit short attention spans, impulsiveness, and aggressive behavior at 1 to 7 years following THI. Those older than 10 showed poor judgment and affective disturbance (Brink, Garrett, Hale, Woo-Sam, & Nickel, 1970). A higher proportion of children versus adults show personality changes following moderate and severe injuries (Shapiro, 1983).

Physical recovery following severe head injury was studied in 344 children and adolescents who were in rehabilitation programs (Brink, Imbus, & Woo-Sam, 1980). Nearly three-fourths of the total sample became ambulatory and capable of self-care; cognitive functioning, however, remained impaired in two-thirds of the patients. Shapiro (1983) contends that independent ambulation can be expected in 70-80% of the THI school-aged population.

With regard to the relationship between age and outcome, Ewing-Cobbs and associates (1985) conclude that:

1. Preschoolers typically exhibit generalized cognitive impairment due to the inherently rapid rate of their cognitive development. This places them at greater risk for developing significant academic delays. Significant attentional, fine and gross motor, intellectual, linguistic, and visuospatial disturbances are common among the brain-injured preschool population.
2. When compared, school-aged children and adolescents show similar neuropsychological profiles following THI. Memory, visual motor, and attentional difficulties are the most common consequences. Beyond the similarities, adolescents will quite often exhibit problems with higher level and more abstract functions such as social judgment, planning, and the ability to use strategies.

Bruce et al. (1978) report that children and adolescents have a greater capacity to survive severe head injuries than adults. This is particularly true for individuals between the ages of 5 and 20 years (Jennett et al., 1979). Children under 15 years who survive are rarely left in a chronic vegetative state; approximately 90% recover to a moderately disabled state within 3 years (Brink et al., 1980; Flach & Malmros, 1972; Stover & Zeiger, 1976).

While Levin et al. (1984) conclude that the outcome of traumatic brain injury is worse in young children as compared to adolescents and adults, Bakay and Glasauer (1980) and Shapiro (1983) consider the long-term outlook for children with severe injuries as better overall. In view of this unresolved controversy and the complicated nature of relating age to outcome, perhaps Rutter et al. (1983) offer the most concise and sensitive appraisal, which is that age differences affect the *rate* of cognitive recovery, the *pattern* of cognitive deficit, and the *extent* of impairment. Based upon the available evidence, it may well be that children and adolescents are more likely to survive head injury and, therefore, tend to fare better than adults with respect to mortality. In terms of morbidity, however, the distinctions are less clear. The differences between the prognoses for these two populations are difficult to generalize because of the interactive influences of numerous variables. In general, it is the capacity to learn and recapture the developmental momentum set forth prior to injury that is the most vulnerable to interruption and not the loss of what has already been mastered. Thus, very young children will be at greater risk for interference of their ability to resume a normal rate and pattern of learning and development (Lehr, 1990a).

Premorbid Characteristics. Intellectual status prior to injury relates positively to outcome following brain damage (Ben-Yishay, Diller, Gerstman, & Gordon, 1970). It is not unreasonable to assume that intellectually brighter students will have more than the average to spare. Rourke et al. (1983) refer to premorbid knowledge as "learned engrams." It has been their contention that the presence or absence of learned engrams following THI greatly affects a child's ability to profit from remediation. Learned engrams are stored systems of information or "pockets of knowledge," which have withstood the effects of injury and, as such, facilitate the recovery process. For example, it is entirely possible for an adolescent to have retained the ability to recognize familiar words, yet be unable to decode unfamiliar words. Overlearning seems to provide some protection against the disruptive consequences of subsequent brain damage (Miller, 1984). Given that brain damage affects the ability to acquire new skills, and well-learned skills tend to be spared, it has been deduced that "better educated" youngsters have a better prognosis for recovery (Rutter, 1981).

Klonoff and Low (1974) found that males were more likely to develop behavioral disturbances (increased irritability) following mild to moderate injuries according to systematic behavioral observations and parental interviews conducted at 1 to 2 years post injury. Secondly, males seemed to be more susceptible than females to Verbal and Performance IQ discrepancies following one-sided lesions (Woods, 1980). In a study of hospitalized survivors of THI, low socioeconomic level was found to be related to frequency of occurrence (Kerr, Kay, & Lassman, 1971). Klonoff (1971) found a disproportionately high number of traumatic head injuries in children who (a) had fathers of a lower economic status, (b) lived in more congested areas, and (c) came from homes with unstable marriages. Psychiatric disorders were found to be more prevalent in children from broken homes and in children whose mothers or fathers experienced psychiatric disorders (Brown, Chadwick, Shaffer, Rutter, & Traub, 1981).

Recovery from THI

In preparation for the return and educational programming of a head-injured student, it is recommended that the professionals responsible become knowledgeable not only about the nature of head injury but about the recovery process as well. School personnel may be expected to provide instructional and ancillary services to students functioning at any point along the recovery continuum. Professionals can find themselves faced with challenges to which they are unaccustomed. An injured student who was once familiar and predictable may reenter the public school system following a period of rehabilitation with a strikingly different intellectual status, physical limitations, numerous learning needs, and a strange and altered personality. Conversely, a former student may reenter appearing fully physically recovered yet be plagued by a series of subtle and troublesome deficits in judgment or by problems with social disinhibition (Boll, 1982; Divack et al., 1985).

Children and adolescents who, due to the severity of their injury, have required hospitalization and a program of rehabilitation are frequently left with cognitive impairment, specific academic problems (Ewing-Cobbs et al., 1985; Heiskanen & Kaste, 1974; Klonoff et al., 1977), memory impairment (Levin & Eisenberg, 1979; Levin, Eisenberg et al., 1982), behavioral disorders (Boll, 1982; Brown et al., 1981), and/or deficits in visual-motor speed (Chadwick, Rutter, Shaffer, & Shrout, 1981; Klonoff & Low, 1974). Depending upon the policies of the rehabilitation facility, the criteria for discharge may vary. Patients are generally discharged once they (a) have plateaued in their physical recovery; (b) are medically stable; (c) are behaviorally manageable; and/or (d) can be transferred to a less restrictive environment, quite possibly home and school. Any one of these criteria may be sufficient enough to warrant a medical discharge. These criteria, set by the medical facility, do not necessarily confirm a student's readiness for a formal school program. Nevertheless, once home, their educational programming becomes the responsibility of the local educational agency. Those who remain medically dependent or seriously characterologically altered are, by law, entitled to public education services (Federal Register, 1977, 1991).

Hagen, Malkmus, and Durham (1981) compiled data on the recovery patterns of over 1,000 patients at the Rancho Los Amigos Hospital in Downey, California. Their aim was to outline the general course of recovery that transpires following traumatic head injury (see Table 11). The product of their efforts is an eight-stage recovery scale which can be used to (a) understand the typical behavioral and cognitive stages of the recovery process; (b) assist professionals, family, and even patients themselves in measuring and anticipating recovery; and (c) aid in the development of treatment programs and strategies for intervention (Szekeres, Ylvisaker, & Holland, 1985).

The rate of recovery can vary dramatically from individual to individual as can the ultimate level each person achieves. Depending upon degree of injury, preaccident developmental status, and post-traumatic treatment, reasonable progress may transport an individual through all stages of recovery within 3-6 months time, whereas another patient with a different profile may never exceed Level II or III. One can readily appreciate the devastating consequences of traumatic head injury as well as the significance of achieving each stage of recovery upon inspection of the Rancho Los Amigos scale. General strategies and instructional objectives that correspond with each behavioral/cognitive level can be found in Chapter 10 (pp. 138–142).

Theories of Recovery

Despite the irreparable damage and scarring that follows traumatic head injury, some degree of recovery almost always occurs (Luria, 1963). Many contend that some functions can be restored, though not necessarily to their original state (Milner, 1974; Schneider, 1979; Woods, 1980). The exact mechanisms by which functions are restored continue to be a matter of scientific study and speculation. The following discussion highlights three commonly regarded mechanisms of recovery.

TABLE 11

RANCHO LOS AMIGOS' LEVELS OF COGNITIVE FUNCTIONING

Early Stages of Recovery
Level I—*No Response*
Patient appears to be in deep sleep and is completely unresponsive to any stimuli presented (coma).

Level II—*Generalized Response*
Patient reacts inconsistently and nonpurposefully to stimuli.

Level III—*Localized Response*
Patient reacts specifically but inconsistently to stimuli; may turn head toward sound or extend hand upon request.

Middle Stages of Recovery
Level IV—*Confused-Agitated*
Patient is in a heightened state of activity; may show aggressive behavior and excessive irritation disproportionate to stimuli; exhibits significantly decreased ability to process information. Speech often reemerges. Short-term memory and selective attention are nonexistent. Patient is unable to perform self-care.

Level V—*Confused, Inappropriate, Nonagitated*
Patient is alert and able to respond to simple commands in a fairly consistent manner; highly distractible; lacks ability to focus and sustain attention; makes inappropriate verbalizations (when motoric speech is not impaired); exhibits severe problems with short-term memory; unable to learn new information. Patient can perform self-help activities with assistance.

Level VI—*Confused-Appropriate*
Patient shows goal-directed behavior and carryover for old skills that have been relearned (toothbrushing, feeding, etc.); continued short-term memory deficits. Long-term memory (recall) is improving. Patient may show inconsistent orientation to time and place; recognizes caretakers and shows some awareness of basic needs.

Late Stages of Recovery
Level VII—*Automatic-Appropriate*
Patient shows increased awareness of self and environment; able to follow a routine schedule with prompts; lacks insight into condition; demonstrates poor judgment and problem-solving skills; unrealistic about future; independent in self-care with supervision; unable to drive a car.

Level VIII—*Purposeful and Appropriate*
Alert and oriented; able to recall and integrate past with recent events; shows carryover for new learning; requires little supervision in carrying out relearned tasks; may continue to show an overall decrease in ability to reason, tolerate stress, and make emergency decisions. Vocational rehabilitation may be indicated.

Inhibition/Disinhibition. The basic premise underlying the theory of inhibition is the assumption that the cellular apparatus needed for the execution of a seemingly lost function, rather than being destroyed by the trauma, is simply in a state of temporary inhibition or inactivity (Luria, 1963). The actual insult may produce temporary physiological disturbances that affect other (not directly damaged) parts of the brain (Miller, 1984). As the condition of this disruption improves, the behavioral impairment (i.e., the suppression of function that has occurred) resolves. For example, the secondary complication of elevated intracranial pressure, once treated and reduced, will parallel the appearance of further recovery. Von Monakow (1914) originally brought forth the concept of *diaschisis* to explain the process of recovery of suppressed or inhibited function. Diaschisis is a kind of postlesional shock which can produce inhibiting effects upon related cerebral areas at some distance from the site of the primary insult (Miller, 1984; Rubens, 1977). This indirect damage causes a functional standstill in otherwise intact areas which generally subsides as the "neural shock" passes (Rourke et al., 1983; Teuber, 1974; West, Deadwyler, Cotman, & Lynch, 1976). Rubens (1977) has speculated that diaschisis may be a function of decreased cerebral blood flow or the release of neurotransmitters. Although the principle of diaschisis has not been well tested, its logic merits strong consideration (Miller, 1984; Teuber, 1974; West et al., 1976).

Luria (1963) defined the general process of inhibition as a reduction of acetylcholine (a neurotransmitter) activity at the synapse caused by an increase in cholinesterase (another neurotransmitter). He was among the first to contend that anticholinesterase drugs such as neostigmine and galanthamine could produce rapid improvements in patients even when prescribed years after the injury (Miller, 1984). Levin (1985) has acknowledged some present-day evidence that the daily ingestion of both lecithin (a dietary source of acetylcholine) and physostigmine (a cholinesterase inhibitor) improves the memory of head-injured persons (Walton, 1982).

Reorganization/Substitution. Underlying the theories of cerebral reorganization (Miller, 1984) or substitution (Luria, 1963) is the premise that not all functions of the brain are forever linked to particular areas of the brain. Damage to one part of the brain may cause other areas to take over the lost function (Bach-y-Rita, 1981). The original damage, however, regardless of the means of reorganization, results in an overall reduction in cognitive mass or efficiency (Rosner, 1974). It may be, for example, that damage to higher (cortical) functions will result in a transfer of their control to a lower (subcortical) level. Hence, the restoration would be of lesser quality (Miller, 1984). Similarly, a function may be taken over by a remote region of the brain, which is often the process used to explain recovery from aphasia (Goldman, 1974a; Luria, 1963; Rourke et al., 1983). For example, language functions damaged by left-sided lesions may be resumed by the right hemisphere (Buffery, 1977; Lezak, 1983). Such reorganization, however, typically reduces the overall capacity of the right hemisphere to carry on its designated functions (Milner, 1974) and may in fact cause a reduction in overall intellectual status (Woods, 1980). The potential for anatomical reorganization is reduced by age and maturity; younger immature brains are more likely to show a transfer of cerebral function than are older more committed brains (Miller, 1984).

Other physiological mechanisms such as denervation supersensitivity (Understedt, 1971), axonal regeneration, collateral sprouting (Schneider, 1979), pruning, and ingrowth (Davis, 1985) have raised intriguing questions about the brain's capacity for neural recovery. Denervation supersensitivity refers to the tendency for neurons which have been deprived of input (denervated) because of damage to acquire an enhanced supersensitivity to neurotransmitters (Goldberger, 1974). Supersensitivity manifests itself as increased electrical activity at the severed area (Rourke et al., 1983). In essence, surviving fibers within a damaged area may come to possess a greater effect than they had prior to damage (Miller, 1984).

Moore (1974) established that axonal growth occurs following damage to the central nervous system. Specifically, when an axon is severed through damage, the part beyond the axon dies. If the remaining or proximal portion continues to live, it may regenerate new axons and terminals (Miller, 1984) (See Figure 8). Usually one outgrowth extends until target recognition and nerve-target association take place; only a few regenerated outgrowths with the proper target and conditions are necessary to reproduce a function (Davis,

71

FIGURE 8

NEURONAL REARRANGEMENTS AFTER BRAIN INJURY

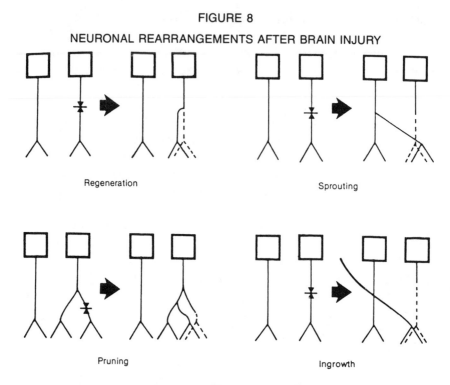

Regeneration   Sprouting

Pruning   Ingrowth

1985). Pruning, like regeneration, is a compensatory response of an injured neuron. Unlike regeneration, the neuronal outgrowth occurs in a different collateral axon which expands to replace the damaged axon (Schneider, 1979). Pruning takes place over several months to years (Davis, 1985).

Collateral sprouting can occur when intact neurons develop sprouts which connect with damaged neurons (Miller, 1984). While there is some evidence to suggest that newly established connections are physiologically functional, they may not necessarily be behaviorally functional (Rourke et al., 1983). Ingrowth is the replacement of damaged fibers by an intact, yet unrelated nerve. Ingrowth occurs over a few weeks to months and does not restore previous neuronal relationships (Davis, 1985). Schneider (1979) hypothesizes that cognitive and behavioral aberrations in humans are the consequence of redirected neuronal growth. Animal studies also cast doubt on the likelihood that regeneration and sprouting reinstate normal function (Matthews, Cotman, & Lynch, 1976; Miller, 1984).

Adaptation. The principle of adaptation following brain injury is most often used to explain long-term recovery in more matured individuals (Miller, 1984). The reattainment of the ability to produce a desired behavior occurs by means of compensation. A different method, thus different neuronal system, is used to overcome the loss of a specific skill. For example, aphasic persons may relearn to communicate by way of compensatory strategies (e.g., by pointing, use of gestures, writing, facial expression, etc.). The use of adaptive strategies and compensatory training to counteract weaknesses is of considerable value in the rehabilitation of head-injured persons (Ben-Yishay et al., 1970; Diller, 1976; Luria, 1963; Rourke et al., 1983).

6

PHYSICAL SEQUELAE OF TRAUMATIC HEAD INJURY: EDUCATIONAL IMPLICATIONS

Motor Deficits

Depending upon the site and extent of damage to the brain, THI can result in varying degrees of motor deficit (Molnar, Jane, & Perrin, 1983). Deficits can range from mild impairment of fine volitional movements to severe paralysis causing a complete loss of functional ability. Physical deficits following brain damage result from lesions to the cortex, brain stem, cranial nerves, or cerebellum (Jennett, 1972). For example, injuries to the motor area of the cortex can cause paralysis and speech disturbances such as stuttering, impairment of lips and tongue movement, or dysfluency (Golden, 1981b). A study by Brink et al. (1980) of 344 children and adolescents following severe injury identified a number of common residual motor deficits including spasticity (38%), ataxia (8%), concomitant spasticity and ataxia (39%), nerve injury (1%), and other (4%) at 1 year post trauma. Ten percent showed significant motor problems. Seventy-three percent achieved motoric independence, 10% were partially dependent, and 17% were totally physically dependent. Other motor residua of THI have been noted as well, such as rigidity, hypotonicity, apraxia, and dysarthria (Jaffe et al., 1985). Table 12 includes a description of the possible neuromotor consequences of THI.

The prognosis for full motor recovery following severe head injury is better than that for a full cognitive recovery (Levin, Benton, & Grossman, 1982; Lishman, 1978). Motor deficits are often temporary

TABLE 12

MOTOR SEQUELAE FOLLOWING THI AND FUNCTIONAL IMPLICATIONS

Dysfunction	Implication
Hemiplegia: Motor paralysis of one side of body	Inhibits movement of arm, face, or leg
Hemiparesis: Motor weakness of one side of body	Limits movement of arm, face, or leg
Hypotonicity: Low muscle tone of trunk or extremities	Prevents initiation of balanced muscle contraction for stability
Rigidity: Resistance to movement in any range	Prevents active movements and good positioning
Spasticity: Inappropriate sustained contraction of muscles	Limits full range of motion. Can lead to contractures. May require drugs or casting
Ataxia: Loss of ability to coordinate smooth movements or steady gait	Limits control of trunk, extremities, and ability to regain balance during movement. To compensate, the patient walks with feet spread apart.
Tremors: Involuntary movements from contractions of opposing muscles	May inhibit fine motor precision of gross motor ability
Apraxia: Problems in planning, organizing, and carrying out sequential movements on command	Prevents deliberate and spontaneous execution of motion or of speech
Dysarthria: Lack of control over automatic oral actions such as chewing, swallowing, and speech	May affect phonation, articulation, feeding, or respiration

and typically resolve long before cognitive recovery is complete (Jaffe et al., 1985). In many rehabilitative settings, youngsters who are recovering from THI may be discharged to home and school prior to the refinement of balance reactions or proper weight shifting and control because they are "functional." For this reason, school personnel need to be prepared to provide an educational extension to the physical rehabilitative process, particularly when such deficits interfere with a child's ability to benefit from special education. Table 13 provides a range of interventions for common physical problems.

TABLE 13

SELECTED INTERVENTIONS FOR COMMON
PHYSICAL PROBLEMS FOLLOWING THI

Problem	Intervention	Study/Source
Hemiparesis	Sensory feedback therapy	Brudny, Korein, Bruce, Grynbaum, Belandres, & Gianutsos, 1979
Failure to propel wheelchair	Mechanical counter of wheelchair revolutions; reinforcement for distance traveled	Grove, 1970
Poor wheelchair transfer	Task analysis, selective reinforcement of small steps toward desired goal	Wood, 1987
Poor head control	Mercury switches attached to cloth collar; musical reinforcement for upright head control	Grove, 1970
Neglect of arm	Automatic auditory and visual feedback for use of arm	Hesse & Friedlander, 1974
Visual neglect	Vertical anchoring line and numbered lines used to guide complete left to right scanning of visual material	Sohlberg & Mateer, 1989
Dysarthria	Ratings of "clear" or "unclear" for speech production; modelling; positive reinforcement and punishment	Ince & Rosenberg, 1973
Dysarthria	Augmentative and alternative communication systems	Marshall, 1989
Swallowing	Praise and attention for swallowing; gradual shaping of chewing and purposeful swallowing	Wood, 1987
Apraxia	Sensory integration therapy	Ayres, 1972
Spasticity	Functional electrical stimulation (FES)	Baker, Parker, & Sanderson, 1983
Severe physical disability	Environmental control systems and switches	Williams, Csongradi, & LeBlanc, 1982
Walking	Tokens awarded for distance traveled; gradual shaping of desired gait	Wood, 1987

Motor functions lost due to brain damage do not return in a reliable and predictable manner. Physical recovery can plateau at any point leaving permanent motor residua behind (Jaffe et al., 1985). Some idea of the process of motor recovery can be gained from an understanding of motor recovery patterns. The functions of lower limbs tend to return sooner and more completely than upper limbs; proximal (trunk) movement returns sooner and more completely than distal (hand, finger) movement (Jennett, 1972). Imagine, as an example, the 13-year-old adolescent who has regained the ability to walk without assistance, but who remains incapable of independent feeding or unable to execute the intricate movements of speech.

In some instances, training in wheelchair locomotion will be necessary (Molnar et al., 1983). A physical therapist may be required to provide the nonambulatory individual with direct training in wheelchair transfers, interclass travel, or in the negotiation of common obstacles, such as restrooms, crowded hallways, cafeterias, elevators, and various terrains (Levin, Eisenberg, & Miner, 1983). Children and adolescents left with visuospatial or perceptual deficits may face unexpected difficulty with body position or spatial orientation. These problems can interfere with the positioning of crutches and canes or wheelchair propulsion, and are likely to warrant special services from a physical or occupational therapist (Ayres, 1972; Evans, 1981; Molnar et al., 1983).

To promote mobility, and decrease hypertonicity, total body movements are preferable to basic range-of-motion exercises (Jaffe et al., 1985). It will be necessary to reestablish movement by emphasizing the more basic and proximal movements first, such as trunk and head control (Evans, 1981). Therapy balls, mats, bolsters, and swimming pools are useful means for developing mobility. The mobility gained during physical therapy can be maintained throughout the day and night by the use of splints and plaster casting (Cusick & Sussman, 1981; Jaffe et al., 1985). Refinement of mild motor deficits can be augmented by means of age-appropriate activities (e.g., balance boards, playing ball, climbing steps, roller skating) or by working in front of a mirror (Jaffe et al., 1985). Evans (1981) has suggested the intermittent use of weighted aids in some cases of cerebellar incoordination. For example, a half-pound weighted cap has proven useful during meals to improve head control as has a weighted vest for ataxic problems when walking.

Traumatically brain-injured children and adolescents may lose functional use of their preferred hand. Consequently, they will need to learn how to perform daily activities with one hand (Avidan, 1977; Evans, 1981), although continued use of the affected hand should be encouraged (Molnar et al., 1983). Repeated verbal reminders and physical restriction of the unaffected limb are apt to promote resistance and frustration and should be avoided (Molnar et al., 1983) in favor of toys, games, functional activities that invite bimanual movement, compensatory aids, and/or visual cues and signals (Evans, 1981; Luria, 1963; Molnar et al., 1983; Rourke et al., 1983).

The transfer of handwriting requirements to the nondominant hand can be a time-consuming and taxing process for older children and adolescents in particular. Students learning to write with their nonpreferred hand will need extra time to complete assignments. Clipboards are helpful for stabilizing paper, and felt tip pens make writing easier. Training in the use of a word processor should be considered when impaired manual functions negatively impact upon a student's educational progress. Step-by-step training in the use of a tape recorder to record lectures or complete written assignments is another viable alternative. Measures should be taken to ensure that extraneous noise does not interfere with the clarity of the taped recording. If a tape recorder is used to record lectures, it should be positioned close to the teacher. As a supplemental aid, a reliable classmate may be assigned to produce a clean photocopy of his/her lecture notes.

While it is often tempting to help disabled individuals perform activities of daily living for the sake of efficiency, it is best that they learn to use adaptive strategies and compensatory aids to perform self-care tasks independently (Rifton Equipment, see Appendix A). Dressing can be made easier with velcro closures, button hooks, long shoe horns, and so forth. When putting on or taking off a coat, for example, hemiplegics should be reminded to put their affected limb in first and to take the affected limb out last. Modified utensils have been developed to make eating easier (Avidan, 1977). These and a variety of other adaptive aids and devices are available for physically limited THI youngsters (Redford, 1980; Sine, Liss, Rousch, & Holcomb, 1977).

The question of whether compensatory training or direct therapy for a motor deficit is the most appropriate intervention is best answered by a physical therapist familiar with both traumatic brain injury and the student requiring services. Regardless of intervention, it is important for therapy to be motivating, functional, and normalized to the extent possible (Luria, 1970a). Age, attitude, time since injury, and degree of deficit need to be taken into consideration when formulating programmatic decisions (Rourke et al., 1983).

Sensory Deficits

Lesions to the primary sensory areas, sensory pathways, or cranial nerves may result in varying degrees of sensory impairment, such as visual field deficits, squinting, defects in color vision, diplopia (double vision), tracking disorders, anosmia (depleted sense of smell), reduced auditory acuity, or sensorineural deafness (Jennett, 1972; Molnar et al., 1983; Rosenthal, Griffith, Bond, & Miller, 1983). A hypersensitivity or hyposensitivity to visual, auditory, olfactory, gustatory, tactile, proprioceptive, and kinesthetic stimuli may also surface following THI (Jaffe et al., 1985). Lesions to secondary visual areas may produce visual agnosias; deficits in figure ground perception, perceptual constancy, and spatial relationships; and reading and writing reversals (Walker, 1989).

Even mild injuries can produce visual impairments such as hemianopsia or field deficit (Jennett, 1972) (see Figure 9). Severe homonymous hemianopsia (loss of half of the visual field on the same side of each eye) may lead to incapacitating reading disability (Anderson & Ford, 1980), as only one half of what is looked at is seen (see Figure 10). Individuals with hemianopsia should be reminded to move their *head* to adjust for their deficit and to compensate with any remaining vision (Avidan, 1977; Caplan, 1982). Students with visual field cuts should be seated in a position that permits strategic alignment of their intact visual field and proper visual access (Rosen & Gerring, 1986). A strategy recommended by Sohlberg and Mateer (1989) for students who experience reading problems as a result of unilateral neglect is to number each paragraph line sequentially at its beginning and end and/or to draw a boldly colored vertical line along the side of the "neglected" margin. In a systematic fashion, each visual cue is gradually faded as performance improves. Verbal reminders to "look left" are also effective.

FIGURE 9

TYPES OF VISUAL FIELD DEFICITS

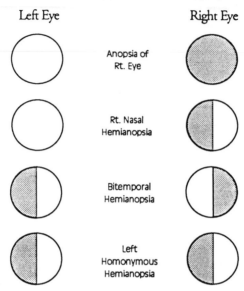

Diplopia is a visual disorder that produces the formation of two unfused images (double vision). Some students may complain that when they read, the words and lines become disorganized. A piece of white cardboard with a cut-out window can be used to expose one line at a time (Avidan, 1977).

Traditional treatments for visual deficits include prism therapy, eye patching, repetitive tabletop activities, and functional exercises (Evans, 1981; Walker, 1989). Vestibular treatments (rigorous rotary activities, rocking, leaning over while seated) are noted in the literature and show some merit for head-injured patients, although conclusive evidence of their efficacy is limited (Walker, 1989).

Cortical blindness is possible but uncommon in children following THI. When it does occur it is usually transient (Jennett & Teasdale, 1981). Optic atrophy from an axonal shearing injury does, however, cause permanent blindness and will require a new reliance upon tactile and auditory input (Scott, Hatten, & Jan, 1979).

Auditory deficits may be related to the head injury or to their subsequent treatment with neurotoxic antibiotics such as strep- tomycin and neomycin (Griffiths, 1979). Auditory deficits are usually

FIGURE 10

EFFECTS OF LEFT HOMONYMOUS HEMIANOPSIA ON READING

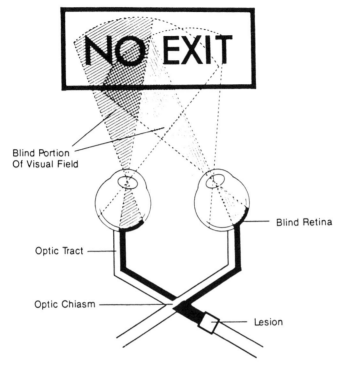

manifested as sensorineural losses (Molnar et al., 1983) and most often affect the high frequency range (Jennett & Teasdale, 1981). Sensorineural deafness is usually caused by damage to either the cochlea or cranial nerve VIII (Liebman, 1986). Ferry and Cooper (1978) recommend that youngsters with bilateral moderate to severe hearing impairment be fitted with hearing aids and receive auditory training and speech/language therapy. In addition to specialized treatments and physical aids (equipment), preferential seating will be necessary for students with auditory deficits.

Seizure Disorder

Although epilepsy is more likely to follow open head injuries than closed head injuries (Golden, Moses, Coffman, Miller, & Strider,

1983), approximately 5% of all closed head injury survivors can be expected to develop epilepsy within 4 years (Jennett, 1972). Seizures following THI are most likely to occur during the first week after the injury ("early epilepsy") or they are delayed for more than 3 months (Jennett, 1972). Early seizures occur more often in children under 5 years of age (Jennett, 1975a) and in both children and adults with more severe injuries (Hauser & Hesdorffer, 1990; Shapiro, 1985). Antiepileptic therapy is usually recommended for patients who continue to have seizures beyond 48 hours (Singer & Freeman, 1978) and is maintained for a period of 1 to 2 seizure-free years (Jennett & Teasdale, 1981). A period of 2 years without seizures is generally required before driving privileges can be granted in the United States (Jennett & Teasdale, 1981). Even after a remission of 2 years, however, there is no guarantee that the risk of seizures ceases for survivors who have had one or more seizures during the first year of their injury (Jennett & Teasdale, 1981). If they remain seizure-free for 3 years, however, most head-injured patients can be 95% certain of avoiding epilepsy (Parker, 1990). Depending upon the complexity of the seizures, drugs such as phenytoin, pheno-barbital, carbamazepine, propranohol, and valproate may be prescribed (Bagby, 1991; Chamovitz, Chorazy, Hanchett, & Mandella, 1985; Horn, 1987). The negative side effects of antiepileptic medications include sedation, speech disturbances, dizziness, and cognitive impairment. Incoordination and weight gain may also result (Bagby, 1991; Smith, 1990). For a classification of seizures and emergency guidelines see Appendix B.

Speech/Language Dysfunction

It is most often the case that severely brain-injured individuals begin to eat before they begin to speak (Jaffe et al., 1985). Speech production can be inhibited by poor muscle tone, poor posture, incoordination, and limited strength, all of which may accompany THI (Jaffe et al., 1985). Dysarthria, which is presumed due to lesions of the left hemisphere (Thompson, 1975), central or peripheral nervous system (Sarno & Levin, 1985), or diffuse cerebral injury (Sarno, 1984), restricts the movements and range of the soft palate, lips, and tongue. Poor phonation skills, which result in a soft and breathy voice, hypernasality, poor articulation, slow rate of speech, and monopitch, are common symptoms of dysarthria (Brookshire, 1978; Jaffe et al., 1985; Sarno, 1980). Apraxia of speech restricts the ability to carry out preplanned, purposeful sequences of oral communication and its imitation (Lezak, 1983). Apraxia frequently occurs as a result of lesions to the premotor area of the cortex (Brookshire, 1978).

Aphasia (the complete or partial impairment of language comprehension, formulation, and use) may result from brain injury (Lezak, 1983), although persistent aphasia following THI is relatively rare (Jennett & Teasdale, 1981). Aphasic symptoms are determined by the area of the cortex which has been damaged (Beaumont, 1983; Goodglass & Kaplan, 1972; Lezak, 1983; Luria, 1973). Aphasia following THI has been found to occur concomitant with such complications as cognitive deficit, memory disorder, faulty reasoning, disorientation, and dyscalculia (loss of the ability to perform arithmetic calculations). Groher, 1977; Hécaen, 1976; Levin, Benton, & Grossman, 1982). Expressive problems may range from temporarily slurred speech to a total loss of communication (U.S. Department of Health, Education, and Welfare, 1979). Anomia (object-naming disturbance) is a common feature of aphasia following closed head injury (Sarno & Levin, 1985). In receptive aphasia (Wernicke's), the ability to comprehend spoken or written language is impaired (Brookshire, 1978; Sarno & Levin, 1985). Global aphasia refers to severe and extensive damage across a number of language functions (Beaumont, 1983). Aphasic individuals are generally better able to comprehend single words and short phrases than lengthy utterances spoken too rapidly. A wide variety of approaches to treatment are used by speech/language pathologists with aphasic patients. Further mention of specific treatment strategies is made in Chapter 10.

Other Complications

Chronic fatigue is a frequent by-product of head trauma (Lezak, 1983). This complication can interfere with a student's ability to resume his/her premorbid pace. Tremendous effort may be necessary to complete the simplest of tasks. Because of limited energy, it may be necessary to reduce courseload or shorten the student's school day. Many THI children and adolescents will do best to return to school on a half-day basis until a reasonable level of endurance has been reestablished (Rosen & Gerring, 1986). Regular, yet unobtrusive, rest periods offset the effects of fatigue. Difficult classes should be scheduled during the student's most productive period of the day.

Because THI can render a youngster hypersensitive to noise (Levin, Grossman, Rose, & Teasdale, 1979) and lower thresholds for stress (Boll, 1982), certain aspects of the typical school day are apt to be particularly taxing, if not overwhelming. Lunchtime, which is generally considered a recess of sorts, may be extremely unsettling. The THI student should be gradually reintroduced to the hectic and overstimulating aspects of the school program. In preparation for the return of a head-injured student whose condition has warranted hospitalization or a program of rehabilitation, it is of benefit to all concerned if key school personnel visit the referring facility prior to patient discharge. Several members of the educational team (e.g., school psychologist, special service providers, guidance counselor, school nurse, special education administrator) should establish contact with rehabilitative personnel (NHIF, 1985). It will be necessary for school staff to become reacquainted with their student and to learn about his/her new physical needs, equipment, and therapy regimens. If this is not possible, rehabilitation specialists and related medical personnel should be invited to participate in planning and eligibility meetings. Some rehabilitation centers may agree to provide a videotape of speech, physical, and occupational therapy routines when meeting is not possible. Special medical and therapeutic recommendations of educational relevance supplied by rehabilitative personnel should be taken seriously and included within the child's individual education program.

7

COGNITIVE SEQUELAE OF TRAUMATIC HEAD INJURY: EDUCATIONAL IMPLICATIONS

The cognitive consequences that follow traumatic head injury are products of the interaction between premorbid anatomical conditions and brain damage (Dikmen, Reitan, & Temkin, 1983). Although various mental aftereffects are associated with THI, cognitive deficits are the most common (Gronwall & Wrightson, 1974; Levin, Benton, & Grossman, 1982). Along with emotional sequelae (see subsequent chapter), cognitive deficits have been found to be more persistent than sensory and motor disorders and generally produce greater social and vocational consequences (Jennett, 1975b; Levin, Benton, & Grossman, 1982). The representation of cognitive deficit following traumatic injury varies from individual to individual, although some generalizations can be made about the functions likely to be disrupted on the basis of research studies and developmental and neurodynamic principles. Intelligence, attention/concentration, language functions, various aspects of memory, abstract reasoning and judgment, academic achievement and new learning, visual motor skills, and perception are highly susceptible to dysfunction. Dikmen et al. (1983) conducted a study of 45 adolescent and adult subjects, the majority of whom had sustained mild to moderate head injuries. The subjects and their matched controls were formally evaluated, initially at 12 months and again at 18 months, by means of the Halstead-Reitan Battery and Trail Making tests. The results supported the following conclusions:

1. Higher level neuropsychological functions seem to be more vulnerable to disruption than lower (subcortical) functions.

85

2. Improvement occurs in complex as well as simple cognitive functions.
3. Cognitive problems in reasoning and conceptualization, flexibility of thought, adaptability to tasks, problem solving, and speed are common early deficits.
4. Cognitive recovery does not necessarily slow down after the first year as was once supposed.
5. Head-injured persons with substantial losses show a relatively greater amount of improvement, due to a greater degree of deficit.
6. Head-injured persons with milder impairments show less improvement and less residual deficit.

Intelligence

Tasks requiring complex integration and immediate problem-solving skills take longer to recover than those that rely upon simple basic skills and past experiences (Dikmen et al., 1983; Mandleberg & Brooks, 1975). Well-learned skills of language, motor, and spatial orientation can assume a psychometrically "average" status within 1-2 years of the injury. Newcombe (1981) has pointed out, however, that standard IQ tests in their tendency to tap acquired knowledge and school learning are likely to underestimate true deficit following brain injury. Levin, Grossman, Rose, and Teasdale (1979) regard the postinjury Verbal IQ as an estimate of premorbid status and the Performance IQ as the better measure of loss and meter of recovery. A study by Chadwick, Rutter, Shaffer, and Shrout (1981) of 25 children with severe head injuries who were matched for controls determined that a variable range of cognitive deficits persisted at 4 months post trauma. Specifically, the *Wechsler Intelligence Scale for Children* (WISC) showed a 10-point decrease in the mean Verbal IQ (VIQ) and a 30-point drop in the mean Performance IQ (PIQ). When these children were reassessed at 1 year post injury, the deficit in VIQ had resolved, whereas the mean PIQ remained 12 points below that for controls. At 2¼ years, the deficit in PIQ remained relatively unchanged.

Children and adolescents with head injury tend to show more pronounced and persistent deficits in Performance versus Verbal IQ. This pattern of intellectual recovery seems to illustrate that well-learned and acquired knowledge returns more quickly and completely than the ability to learn new skills and solve problems (Brooks & Aughton, 1979; Hebb, 1942). Viewed another way, visual-perceptual and visual-motor deficits are more resistant to recovery than are verbal abilities (Chadwick, Rutter, Shaffer, & Shrout, 1981).

Attention/Concentration

Problems with attention and concentration are common following brain damage (Lezak, 1983). Head-injured children who had been experiencing attentional deficits or problems with concentration prior to the injury are likely to experience an exaggeration of these disturbances after the trauma (Kolb & Whishaw, 1980; Szekeres et al., 1985). Attentional deficits refer to distractibility or impaired ability for focused behavior (Lezak, 1983). Concentration problems are the result of an attentional disturbance. Both attention and concentration are prerequisites for mental tracking. Gronwall and Sampson (1974) contend that information processing deficits following head injury may be attributed to an alteration in arousal level. A short attention span, inflexible thought processes, and stimulus-bound behavior (Lezak, 1983; Szekeres et al., 1985) can seriously compromise academic progress, not to mention social appeal. For example, a youngster may have difficulty on tasks requiring the manipulation of several variables at once. Due to delimited attention, the child is apt to form a simplified perception of the task and produce a simplified response. Casual conversations with stimulus-bound individuals are likely to reflect their perseverative tendencies and inability to shift mental sets. Their conversation is often irrelevant and disorganized because they are unable to grasp the theme and remain oriented (Goodglass & Kaplan, 1979). An accurate identification of the basis for apparent attention or concentration deficits is a necessary prerequisite to proper treatment. What sometimes appear to be attentional deficits and distractibility are often manifestations of an underlying visuo-spatial, perceptual, or constructional disorder (Newcombe, 1981). The specific nature of the deficit needs to be identified, otherwise remedial efforts will be unnecessarily misdirected (Levin, Eisenberg, & Miner, 1983).

Language Functions

Aphasic disorder produced by head injury in children differs from that found in adolescents. Initially, the child's recovery is characterized by mutism with relatively well-preserved language comprehension (Levin et al., 1983). Word-finding difficulty (anomia) existing concurrently with fluent speech and impaired comprehension is common during the early stage of recovery in adolescents and adults. Virtually all aphasic victims of THI show some degree of word-finding difficulty (Goodglass & Kaplan, 1979; Sarno & Levin, 1985). Verbal reasoning and verbal memory functions are often impaired (Baxter, Cohen, & Ylvisaker, 1985). The speed and ease of verbal production (fluency), reading comprehension, and writing are also sensitive to the effects of THI (Lezak, 1983). Both children and adolescents may have difficulty with the mechanics of writing because they are unable to (a) recall letter-forming movements, (b) remember how words are spelled (symbol recall), or (c) combine words into sentences (syntax) (Goodglass & Kaplan, 1979). Auditory comprehension may be impaired in a global or highly selective manner, whereby classes of words (e.g., colors, numbers, or prepositions) are exclusively affected (Gardner, Strub, & Albert, 1975; Geschwind & Fusillo, 1966).

Strategic lesions to the language regions of the left hemisphere of right-handers (those most likely to have language mediated by the left hemisphere) lead to impairment of language functions with few exceptions (Goodglass & Kaplan, 1979; Levin, 1985). Levin estimated that approximately two-thirds of the individuals who suffer significant expressive or receptive language deficits following severe closed head injuries recover fully or at least improve to the point where only word-finding or word-naming ability is impaired. Approximately one-third are left with severe language deficits.

Memory

Disorders of memory are widely held as the most common neuropsychological consequences of THI and are among the most persistent (Levin, 1985). Russell (1932) introduced the term *post traumatic amnesia* to highlight the significance of memory loss as an index of severity. The vulnerability of the temporal lobes and the diffuse white matter shearing that characterizes closed head injuries are presumed responsible for the emergence of residual memory disturbances (Alexander, 1984; Pang, 1985).

Many terms are used in the literature to distinguish the different types of memory. Wilson (1987) identifies eight types of memory:

short- and long-term memory; verbal and non-verbal memory; episodic and semantic memory; and visual and auditory memory. Short-term memory (STM), also referred to as primary or "working" memory, has the capacity to hold up to seven chunks of information. The descriptor "short-term" implies retention of up to one minute (Levin, 1985). Long-term or secondary memory refers to the storage and retrieval of information held beyond one minute (Wilson & Moffat, 1984). With recovery, the facility for retrieving old (long-term) memories returns first, followed by memory for events closer in time to the injury (Goodglass & Kaplan, 1979; Lezak, 1983). Individuals rendered unconscious by head trauma commonly experience a loss of memory for events preceding the injury (retrograde amnesia), sometimes amounting to hours or days before the accident (Ewing-Cobbs, Fletcher, & Levin, 1985; Goodglass & Kaplan, 1979; Lezak, 1983). Disturbances in new learning can coexist with an intact short-term memory.

Memory efficiency has been found to be negatively related to coma duration (i.e., severity of injury) but unrelated to age and education (Hannay, Levin, & Grossman, 1979; Levin et al., 1982). Verbal memory deficits were found to persist as long as 10 years after the injury in approximately 25% of a sample of moderately to severely injured school-aged children (Gaidolfi & Vignolo, 1980).

Highly circumscribed memory deficits can follow THI. For example, some head-injured youngsters may be able to recount their personal experiences and temporal relationships remarkably well (episodic memory), but be unable to recall general information, such as a knowledge of symbols, concepts, or the name of the president of the United States (semantic memory). Memory deficits may be selectively manifested as impairments in visual recognition (Hannay et al., 1979; Levin, Grossman, & Kelley, 1976; Wilson, 1987), verbal memory, visual memory (Levin, Eisenberg et al., 1982), auditory memory or motor skill learning (Corkin, 1968). Memory deficits often persist and interfere with academic progress, despite the recovery of "average" intelligence (Levin, Benton, & Grossman, 1982).

Patten (1982) investigated the process of memory recovery in 50 patients with memory problems due to right-hemisphere, left-hemisphere, or bilateral lesions and determined that:

1. Recent memory tended to be more impaired than rote memory.

2. Over half of those studied experienced deficits in rote memory.
3. Recent memory deficits accompanied rote memory impairment.
4. Patients with right-hemisphere damage did better with verbal memory tasks.
5. Patients with left-hemisphere damage did better with visual memory tasks.

Conceptual Functions, Abstract Reasoning, and Judgment

Conceptual dysfunction is not easily associated with lesions to a particular cortical site as are some language functions (Lezak, 1983). Rather, conceptual dysfunction is associated with brain damage per se (Luria, 1966). Lezak (1983) clarified this phenomenon in her explanation of the interactional nature of conceptual functioning: Conceptual functioning requires (a) an intact perceptual system; (b) a store of accessible memories; (c) intact cortical and subcortical neural pathways; (d) the capacity to process two or more events simultaneously; (e) an intact output modality to put thoughts into action; and (f) an intact feedback system that permits monitoring and modulation. The inability to think abstractly (i.e., the tendency toward concrete thinking) makes it difficult to distinguish the relevant from irrelevant and essential from nonessential elements. Individuals who sustain moderate to severe brain injury and those with diffuse damage tend to do poorly on measures of abstract thinking (Lezak, 1983). They may have difficulty understanding categories, generalizing, or applying rules of grammar, math, and conventional behavior. They may make inappropriate or offensive remarks and frequently miscommunicate their intentions (Haarbauer-Krupa, Henry, Szekeres, & Ylvisaker, 1985).

Academic Achievement/New Learning

Scholastic achievement may be affected by mild, moderate, and severe head injuries (Boll, 1982; Goldstein & Levin, 1985; Richardson, 1963; Rimel et al., 1981). In a follow-up assessment of THI children (less than 12 years old) at 2 years post trauma, a high rate of residual reading disability was found (Shaffer, Bijur, Chadwick, & Rutter, 1980). Of the 88 children studied, 55% showed a reading level that was 1 year below grade-level expectancy. Thirty-three percent were more than 2 years behind. In a later study of 18 children and adolescents, the degree of residual reading deficit ranked second to significant impairment in arithmetic functions (Goldstein & Levin, 1985). The calculation disturbance was not related to the severity of the injury, nor was it limited to patients with significantly impaired IQs. Hécaen (1976) studied 16 school-aged children with aphasia and found that impairment in the ability to perform arithmetic operations was a common accompaniment.

The young child who has not yet acquired reading skills may experience difficulty when the development of such skill is expected. Evidence of academic dysfunction may take several months or more to surface (Sohlberg & Mateer, 1989). Academic proficiency will often be inconsistent. For example, math problems may be computed correctly one day and incorrectly the next.

Despite achievement test data that suggest grade-level appropriateness, residual memory impairments, problems with new learning, and reduced motor speed often remain (Chadwick, Rutter, Shaffer, & Shrout, 1981). Naturally, these residua will have a detrimental and cumulative effect upon school performance. As stated elsewhere, achievement test scores of head-injured pupils must be interpreted as different from scores of students whose brain function has not been artificially and dramatically altered. At best, achievement levels following a head injury become estimates of retention and recall; they no longer retain their predictive value (Baxter et al., 1985).

Perception

Visual-motor and visual-perceptual problems are also common in head-injured children and adolescents. Such problems may show up as configural distortions, misperceptions, or problems with directionality (Lezak, 1983). Both left- and right-hemisphere-damaged individuals tend to make significantly more errors on the side contralateral to the lesion (Lezak, 1983). Levin and Eisenberg (1979) found that visuospatial deficits, as measured by the construction of three-dimensional block designs and Bender performances, were present in nearly one-third of the closed head-injured children they studied. Poor attention to detail, slow visual-motor dexterity, and poor part-to-whole conceptualization are recognized sequelae of THI

(Chadwick, Rutter, Shaffer, & Shrout, 1981; Klonoff & Low, 1974; Klonoff, Low, & Clark, 1977; Levin et al., 1977; Lezak, 1983).

While specific high-level perceptual deficits (i.e., agnosias) have been found in individuals after penetrating (open) head injuries (Benton, 1979b), facial discrimination disturbances in particular have been found among mild to severe cases of closed head injury (Levin et al., 1977). Lesions in the association areas adjacent to each of the three primary sensory areas can compromise the ability to recognize stimuli in spite of normal primary sensory functions (Goodglass & Kaplan, 1979). With *visual agnosia,* objects can be seen and described but not recognized. Individuals suffering from visual agnosia must rely upon tactile cues to supplant recognition. *Prosopagnosia* is the loss of the ability to recognize faces by way of visual perception (Levin et al., 1977). Individuals suffering from prosopagnosia must rely upon voice to identify unrecognizable people (Goodglass & Kaplan, 1979). *Tactile agnosia* prevents an individual from recognizing objects by touch alone. *Auditory agnosia* interferes with the ability to recognize the nature of sounds perceived, despite normal auditory acuity (Goodglass & Kaplan, 1979).

8

PSYCHIATRIC, PSYCHOSOCIAL, AND BEHAVIORAL SEQUELAE OF TRAUMATIC HEAD INJURY: EDUCATIONAL IMPLICATIONS

Determinants of Outcome

As a consequence of THI, the risk of psychiatric and psychosocial complication is substantially increased (Barin et al., 1985; Rutter, 1981). Tables 14 and 15 identify the range of behavioral sequelae that can accompany mild, moderate, and severe head injuries. The relationship between psychiatric consequences and brain injury, however, is not necessarily causal (Rutter, 1981). Although psychiatric disorder is most likely the result of abnormal neuro-physiological activity and is influenced to some extent by the nature of injury and medical condition, other variables may account for the development of emotional and behavioral problems. Rutter (1981) offers five equally plausible determinants of psychiatric problems following THI:

1. *Constitutional factors*. The influences of psychosocial stress and constitution, for example, can produce psychiatric disorders. Postinjury disturbance may be an extension of a premorbid condition.
2. *Secondary handicaps*. Because THI frequently produces physical disability or physical change, psychological sequelae are often a function of the acquired physical handicaps.
3. *Low IQ*. Because THI frequently results in intellectual impairment, emotional and behavioral problems may stem from a low IQ rather than, or in addition to, brain damage.

93

TABLE 14

PSYCHIATRIC AND PSYCHOSOCIAL SEQUELAE OF MILD THI

Behavioral Manifestation	Source
Headache	Binder & Rattok, 1989; Boll, 1982; Cartlidge & Shaw, 1981; Levin, Benton, & Grossman, 1982
Dizziness	Binder & Rattok, 1989; Boll, 1982; Cartlidge & Shaw, 1981; Levin et al., 1982
Fatigue	Binder & Rattok, 1989; Boll, 1982; Levin et al., 1982; Lezak, 1983
Irritability	Levin et al., 1982; Cartlidge & Shaw, 1981
Anxiety	Cartlidge & Shaw, 1981; Levin & Grossman, 1978
Sleep disturbance	Boll, 1982; Levin et al., 1982; Lishman, 1973
Hypochondriacal concern	Levin et al., 1982; Levin & Grossman, 1978; Lishman, 1973
Hypersensitivity to noise	Levin et al., 1982; Lezak, 1983
Photophobia	Levin et al., 1982
Memory problems	Binder & Rattok, 1989; Boll, 1982; Levin et al., 1982; Rimel, Giordani, Barth, Boll, & Jane, 1981
Attention deficit	Rimel et al., 1981
Poor judgment	Rimel et al., 1981; Rosen & Gerring, 1986

4. *Predisposition to disturbance.* The cause of brain injury and subsequent psychological disturbance may be related. For example, disruptive children of limited intelligence may be predisposed to head injury because they are more likely to engage in unsafe and injury-prone behavior.
5. *Psychosocial variables.* Psychosocial deprivation may increase the likelihood of brain injury as well as influence outcome.

The significance of these and other neurophysiological and premorbid variables upon the rate and type of psychiatric disturbance is discussed in the following sections.

Nature of Injury

Extent of Injury. Evidence shows that severe head injury increases the likelihood of psychiatric disturbance, whereas mild injury does not (Rutter, 1981). In a prospective study of children with mild and severe head injuries, it was found that children with severe head injuries developed psychiatric disorders three times as often as their controls and those who were mildly injured (Brown, Chadwick, Shaffer, Rutter, & Traub, 1981; Rutter, 1981). Three groups of children were studied: (a) those with severe head injuries, (b) those with mild head injuries, and (c) control subjects with orthopedic injuries alone. Assessment of each child's preaccident behavior was extrapolated from parent interviews conducted after the accident and from teacher questionnaires. All three groups were followed for 27 months. Standardized assessment took place at 4, 12, and 27 months. Although the rates of behavioral disorder prior to injury were similar across groups, within 4 months the rate of disorder significantly increased in the group with severe head injuries. Furthermore, the rate of disorder in the severely head-injured group remained well above that of the control group throughout the 27-month course.

Laterality/Site. Rutter, Graham, and Yule (1970) found that psychiatric disturbance was significantly more common in cases of bilateral injury than it was when damage was confined to one side of the brain. In adults, and frequently in older adolescents, affective (mood) disorders are often associated with right-hemisphere lesions, particularly if the frontal lobes are involved (Lishman, 1978). Flor-Henry (1979), for example, noted an increased tendency for depression following lesions to the right frontal and left parieto-occipital areas. For the most part, the locus of dysfunction responsible for psychiatric sequelae is less consistent and less marked in children (Ritvo, Ornitz, & Walter, 1970; Rutter et al., 1970). There is also a general tendency for psychiatric disorders to occur when lesions are complicated by epilepsy or by abnormal EEG discharges (i.e., active physiological disturbance) (Rutter et al., 1970). Shaffer, Chadwick, and Rutter (1975) found that psychiatric disorders are also more common in children who develop late epilepsy.

TABLE 15

PSYCHIATRIC AND PSYCHOSOCIAL SEQUELAE OF MODERATE
AND SEVERE THI

Behavioral Manifestation	Source
Hoarding	Boll, 1982
Boredom	Boll, 1982; Oddy, Humphrey, & Uttley, 1978b; Weddell, Oddy, & Jenkins, 1980
Denial of problems	Barin, Hanchett, Jacob, & Scott, 1985; Blazyk, 1983; Boll, 1982; Goethe & Levin, 1984; Weinstein & Lyerly, 1968
Euphoria	Benton, 1979b; Boll, 1982; Jennett, 1972
Irritability	Boll, 1982; Goethe & Levin, 1984; McKinlay, Brooks, & Bond, 1981; Richardson, 1963; Thompsen, 1974
Social withdrawal	Benton, 1979b; Boll, 1982; Levin, Eisenberg, & Miner, 1983; Levin & Grossman, 1978
Suspiciousness	Boll, 1982
Hostility, aggression	Boll, 1982; Goethe & Levin, 1984; Levin & Grossman, 1978
Lack of foresight	Boll, 1982; Goethe & Levin, 1984
Anxiety	Boll, 1982; Cartlidge & Shaw, 1981; Goethe & Levin, 1984; Richardson, 1963
Restlessness	Boll, 1982; Levin, Eisenberg, & Miner, 1983; Thompsen, 1974
Delusions of grandiosity	Boll, 1982; Levin, Benton, & Grossman, 1982
Sleep disturbances	Boll, 1982; Newcombe, 1981; Symonds, 1940
Social crudeness	Goethe & Levin, 1984; Lezak, 1978; Rutter, 1981; Rutter, Chadwick, & Shaffer, 1983
Silliness	Barin et al., 1985; Boll, 1982; Jennett, 1972; Levin & Grossman, 1978
Disinhibition	Boll, 1982; Burgess & Wood, 1990; Jennett, 1972; Rutter, 1981; Weddell et al., 1980
Reduced initiative	Goethe & Levin, 1984; Jennett, 1972; Lezak, 1978; Oddy & Humphrey, 1980; Rosen & Gerring, 1986

(continued)

TABLE 15

CONTINUED

Behavioral Manifestation	Source
Blunting of emotion	Boll, 1982; Levin & Grossman, 1978
Increased affection	Weddell et al., 1980
Decreased libido	Barin et al., 1985; Blazyk, 1983; Boll, 1982
Lability of affect	Boll, 1982; Jennett, 1972; Levin & Grossman, 1978
Depression	Barin et al., 1985; Benton, 1979b; Blazyk, 1983; Cartlidge & Shaw, 1981; Goethe & Levin, 1984; Levin & Grossman, 1978
Disorientation	Benton, 1979b; Levin & Grossman, 1978; Rosen & Gerring, 1986
Stubbornness	Thompsen, 1974
Dependency	Blazyk, 1983; Newcombe, 1981; Weddell et al., 1980
Hypersensitivity to noise	Benton, 1979b; Levin, Grossman, James, Rose, & Teasdale, 1979
Impaired attention/ concentration	Benton, 1979b; Brink et al., 1970; Lezak, 1978
Fatigue	Lezak, 1983; Brooks & McKinlay, 1983; Richardson, 1963
Excitability	Brooks & McKinlay, 1983; Lezak, 1983
Changed sex drive	Blumer & Benson, 1975; Boller & Frank, 1981; Lezak, 1978; Symonds, 1940
Violent tendencies	Barin et al., 1985; Burgess & Wood, 1990
Self-centeredness	Oddy, Humphrey, & Uttley, 1978b
Self-doubt	Barin et al., 1985; Lezak, 1983
Posttraumatic psychosis or neurosis	Cartlidge & Shaw, 1981; Levin, Benton, & Grossman, 1982
Confabulation	Levin, Benton, & Grossman, 1982; Weinstein & Lyerly, 1968

HEAD INJURY IN CHILDREN AND ADOLESCENTS

Premorbid Factors

Age at injury bears no relationship upon the potential for psychiatric risk (Chadwick, Rutter, Thompson, & Shaffer, 1981; Levin, Ewing-Cobbs, & Benton, 1984; Shaffer et al., 1975). Shapiro (1983) has made the point, however, that personality changes occur more often in moderately and severely injured children than in adults. Perhaps this seeming contradiction is brought into focus by the work of Brink et al. (1970) who identified a relationship between age and *type* of behavioral manifestation. Children under 10 years of age were found to exhibit signs of hyperactivity, a short attention span, impulsive behavior, and aggressiveness, whereas those older than 10 years showed affective disturbances and poor judgment. With respect to the relationship between residual psychiatric disturbance and age, Rutter (1981) contends that although there are no significant differences in the likelihood of psychiatric disorder in THI children versus THI adults, the effects of the disturbance are different, as is the rate of recovery, which seems to be marginally more rapid in children.

The premorbid personality of traumatically brain-damaged individuals has been found to influence the quality of adjustment and amount of gain they make (Lishman, 1973), in that premorbid personality characteristics are often exaggerated by brain injury (Lezak, 1983). The existence of preinjury behavior problems substantially increases the likelihood of emotional disorders following the injury (Brown et al., 1981). Impulsive, overactive youngsters, who by nature are more inclined to participate in dangerous activities, are at greater risk for head injury and more likely to develop psychiatric complications (Burton, 1968; Rutter, 1981). Similarly, psychiatric disorder is more common in brain-damaged children from broken homes and in those whose mothers exhibited an emotional disturbance (Rutter et al., 1970). Social disadvantage, marital discord, and parental mental disorder further increase the risk for psychiatric problems following head injury (Shaffer et al., 1975).

Low IQ prior to injury and premorbid reading difficulties have been associated with an increased potential for behavior and emotional problems (Brown et al., 1981; Seidel, Chadwick, & Rutter, 1975). Klonoff and Low (1974) found males to be more vulnerable to increased irritability following injury, whereas personality changes were found to occur proportionally in males and females.

In sum, severity of injury, type of damage, premorbid behavior, psychosocial status, parental emotional stability, and premorbid intellectual and academic status seem to affect the *rate* at which psychiatric disorders occur. Site and laterality of lesion, age at injury, and sex are associated with the *type* of disorder that follows. Although brain injury per se is a significant cause of psychiatric disorder following THI, it is but one of many neurological and non-neurological influences (Ewing-Cobbs et al., 1985; Rutter et al., 1983).

Psychological Adjustment

Social and emotional functioning may deteriorate over time in response to a personal awareness of lost cognitive, social, and/or physical functions (Fordyce, Roueche, & Prigatano, 1983; Lezak, 1983). Many children and adolescents can recognize changes in their ability to perform tasks that were once easy. Young children may try to deny their inabilities by taking dangerous risks; older children and adolescents may develop an apathetic attitude, become easily angered, or withdraw from social interaction (Barin et al., 1985; Fordyce et al., 1983). For school-aged individuals, peer relationships are often compromised following a head injury (Barin et al., 1985). Old friends may lose interest and patience, forcing the THI child or adolescent into isolation or towards relationships with much younger companions in search of acceptance and developmental or emotional parity. The affective and behavioral complications associated with cerebral trauma, such as poor impulse control, aggression, and disinhibition, make old friendships difficult to sustain (Barin et al., 1985). For adolescents, normal development towards individuation and independence may be disrupted or even reversed (Blazyk, 1983; Lehr, 1990a). Although age-relevant issues of autonomy, sexuality, self-image, identity, and achievement remain, the capacity for resolving these issues may be permanently lessened by the neurobehavioral consequences of severe head injury. To adolescents, the loss of driving privileges because of neuropsychological deficits or the threat of seizures is a very real and persistent reminder of lost independence (Blazyk, 1983; Barin et al., 1985; Jennett, 1983a).

Both family and head-injured member need an honest yet sensitive explanation of the psychological findings and a careful report of functional strengths and weaknesses (Lezak, 1983). When sharing information, it is best to be honest yet sensitive and respectful of their need to strive and hope. After all, it is impossible to predict with absolute accuracy what and how much change will take place as the brain recovers or the degree to which environmental variables (therapy, family, motivation) will influence outcome. The social and psychological ties of the family, disrupted dreams, the sudden dependency of the head-injured member, and a pervasive sense of loss render families of THI individuals vulnerable to emotional stress and exasperation (Lezak, 1978). Even subtle changes in the cognitive, physical, affective, or behavioral tone of their child can produce significant adjustment reactions on the part of the parent, Self-centeredness, apathy, impulsivity, irritability, and loss of initiative are but a few of the consequences likely to make family adjustment difficult (Bond, 1983; Oddy, Humphrey, & Uttley, 1978a).

Denial is a common reaction to the unexpected impact of the trauma (Barin et al., 1985). Unrealistically high expectations about recovery can compound problems arising from the THI individual's changed personality. Low expectations coupled with overprotection can be sustained by guilt or fear of social criticism (Buck, 1968; Malone, 1977). Depression, too, is a common response among injured persons and their families (Blazyk, 1983; Lezak, 1983). Relatives who were particularly close to the injured child and those who feel restricted by a sudden dependency are at risk for depression (Lezak, 1978). It is not uncommon for those affected to entertain thoughts of suicide. Some may attempt to dull the pain with alcohol or drugs (Bond, 1983; Lezak, 1978). Bond contends that most family members take between 1 and 2 years to develop a realistic perspective of the disability and nearly as long to develop the means to cope.

9

ASSESSMENT OF TRAUMATICALLY HEAD-INJURED CHILDREN AND ADOLESCENTS

The placement of assessment as one of the final chapters should not be read as an indication that assessment is without prominence in the treatment paradigm. Given that critical questions regarding educational placement, eligibility for related services, and appropriate instructional goals will be answered by the findings of formal evaluations, the significance of precise and frequent appraisals should be quite clear. Its placement here is intended to highlight the importance of conducting formal assessments *after* having developed an appreciation for traumatic brain injury and the features that distinguish THI individuals from other exceptional learners.

Unlike the many referrals submitted to educational evaluation teams which question the presence of brain dysfunction, the confirmation of underlying brain pathology is not central to the evaluation of children known to have sustained brain damage. The critical questions are more likely to be qualitative and practical in nature (e.g., To what extent has this individual recovered? Which functions continue to show impairment and to what degree? What strategies are likely to promote recovery and normalization?) The degree to which traditional psychometric tests are able to measure these dimensions of dysfunction is, however, limited. The validity of standardized instruments and the degree to which they are capable of yielding unbiased and comparable results becomes immeasurably altered when applied to traumatically brain-damaged individuals (Chadwick & Rutter, 1983; Lezak, 1983).

The processes of test administration and interpretation following traumatic brain injury should be undertaken from a neuropsychological purview, that is, with full consideration of the precariousness of cerebral conditions, specific neuropsychological variables, and a sensitivity to the range of aberrations possible. The potential for rapid change makes frequent assessment necessary. Variables such as the type, extent, and site of injury; age; time since injury; and premorbid functioning will influence the assessment process. Given the range of possible consequences, a variety of instruments should be used to ensure examination of the most susceptible of functions (Golden & Mariush, 1986). Boll (1982), Hynd and Orbzut (1981), Lezak (1983), Rourke et al. (1983), and others have collectively identified these functions (see Table 16). Table 17 provides a list of formal procedures for examining each vulnerable construct. Unless the examination process is geared to elicit evidence of possible dysfunction, serious deficits are apt to be ignored (Eson & Bourke, 1980).

To permit a finer analysis of individual abilities and capture the quality of spared and impaired functions following traumatic brain injury, it may be necessary to modify standard administration procedures (Kaplan, 1988). Otherwise, the nature and effectiveness of the strategies employed by the examinee en route to a solution will be lost to the superficiality of simple binary scoring (i.e., credit or no credit). Careful assessment of error patterns, the ability to make conceptual shifts, dexterity, modality preferences, and problem-solving strategies provides the kind of insight needed to appreciate fully *how* it is that underlying processes are affected and the extent to which recovery is occurring. With this information, practical treatment recommendations are more easily generated. Because fatigue is a chronic by-product of THI, frequent rests or shortened evaluative sessions are recommended (Baxter et al., 1985; Lezak, 1983). If test directions are inadequate due to the examinee's residual sensory, verbal, or motor impairment, formal instructions should be adapted with changes in format explicitly documented for purposes of replication (Lezak, 1983; Sattler, 1982).

In order to satisfy the requirements for both quantitative and qualitative data, Lezak (1983) suggests using a double scoring procedure. A functional score is obtained by following standardization rules. The second score is a combination of standardized score plus raw score points earned upon testing the limits. The disparity

TABLE 16

FUNCTIONS TO BE EXAMINED FOLLOWING THI

Intelligence
- verbal
- nonverbal

Attention/Concentration
- visual
- auditory

Communication
- spoken vs. written
- receptive vs. expressive
- speech vs. language

Memory
- short-term and long-term
- verbal and nonverbal
- episodic and semantic
- visual and auditory

New Learning Ability

Abstract Reasoning and Judgment

Orientation
- personal
- spatial
- temporal

Manual Dexterity/Laterality
- left vs. right
- lateral dominance

Academic Achievement

Personality/Adjustment

Perception (visual, auditory, tactile functions)
- sensory
- visual-motor

Behavior
- among peers, family, strangers
- home, school, community

---

provides an estimate of lost ability. When testing the limits, special attention should be paid to how problems are tackled and the ways in which performance is enhanced by means of stimulus and response adjustments (Cicerone & Tupper, 1986). What strategies does the child employ to compensate for his or her physical, cognitive, and sensory deficits? Is performance heightened by visual prompts, verbal directives, or demonstration? How does increased response time or a multiple choice format affect performance?

103

TABLE 17

FORMAL ASSESSMENT PROCEDURES AND TECHNIQUES FOR CHILDREN
AND ADOLESCENTS FOLLOWING THI

Intelligence
British Ability Scales (Elliott, Murray, & Pearson, 1983)
Columbia Mental Maturity Scale (Burgemeister, Blum, & Lorge, 1972)
Differential Ability Scales (Elliot, 1990)
Kaufman Assessment Battery for Children (Kaufman & Kaufman, 1983)
Leiter International Performance Scale (Leiter, 1969)
Nonverbal Test of Cognitive Ability (Johnson & Boyd, 1981)
Pictorial Test of Intelligence (French, 1964)
Raven's Standard Progressive Matrices (Raven, 1986)
Stanford-Binet Intelligence Scale: Fourth Edition (Thorndike, Hagen, & Sattler, 1986)
Wechsler Adult Intelligence Scale - Revised (Wechsler, 1981)
Wechsler Intelligence Scale for Children - III (Wechsler, 1991)
Wechsler Preschool and Primary Scale of Intelligence - Revised (Wechsler, 1989)
Woodcock-Johnson Psycho-Educational Battery—Revised (WJ-R): Tests of Cognitive
   Ability (Woodcock & Johnson, 1989)

Attention/Concentration
Freedom from Distractibility (Wechsler scales)
Matching Familiar Figures Test (Campbell, 1976)
Paced Auditory Serial Addition Test (Gronwall & Sampson, 1974)
Rhythm subtest (Luria-Nebraska Neuropsychological Battery - Children's Revision)
   (LNNB-C) (Golden, Purisch, & Hammeke, 1985)
Seashore Rhythm Test (Halstead-Reitan Battery) (Halstead, 1947)

Communication
Boston Diagnostic Aphasia Examination (Goodglass & Kaplan, 1972)
Communicative Abilities in Daily Living (Holland, 1980)
Controlled Oral Word Association (Benton, Hamsher, Varney, & Spreen, 1983)
Expressive One-Word Vocabulary Test - Revised (Gardner, 1990)
Multilingual Aphasia Examination (Benton & Hamsher, 1978)
Peabody Picture Vocabulary Test - Revised (Dunn, 1981)
Porch Index of Communicative Ability (Porch, 1967)
Selective Reminding Test (Buschke & Fuld, 1974)
Test of Adolescent Word Finding (German, 1990)
Test for Auditory Comprehension of Language - Revised (Carrow-Woolfolk, 1985)
Test of Written Language - Second Ed. (Hammill & Larsen, 1988)
Token Test for Children (DiSimoni, 1978)
Vocabulary subtest (Wechsler scales)

Memory
Benton Visual Retention Test (Benton, 1974)
Digit Span subtest (Wechsler scales)
Information subtest (Wechsler scales)

(continued)

TABLE 17

CONTINUED

Rivermead Behavioral Memory Test - Revised (Wilson, Cockburn, & Braddeley, 1985)
Sentence Memory Test (Benton, 1965)
Short Term and Long Term Memory clusters (WJ-R)
Visual Aural Digit Span Test (Koppitz, 1977)
Wechsler Memory Scale - Revised (Wechsler, 1987)

New Learning Ability
Category Test (Reitan, 1959)
Performance Scale (Wechsler scales)
Reitan-Modified Halstead Category Test (Kimura, 1981)
Selective Reminding Test (Buschke & Fuld, 1974)
Serial Digit Learning (Benton, Hamsher, Varney, & Spreen, 1983)
Wisconsin Card Sorting Test (Grant & Berg, 1980)

Abstract Reasoning/Judgment
British Ability Scales (Elliott, Murray, & Pearson, 1983)
Category Test (Reitan, 1959)
Comprehension subtest (Wechsler scales)
Matrix Analogies Test (Naglieri, 1985)
Similarities subtest (Wechsler scales)
Wisconsin Card Sorting Test (Grant & Borg, 1980)

Orientation
• Children's Orientation and Amnesia Test (Ewing-Cobbs et al., 1984)
• Galvestion Orientation and Amnesia Test (Levin, O'Donnell, & Grossman, 1979)
Personal Orientation Test (Benton et al., 1983)
Right-Left Orientation Test (Benton et al., 1983)
Spatial Orientation Memory Test (Wepman & Turaids, 1975))
Standardized Road Map Test of Direction Sense (Money, 1976)
Temporal Orientation Test (Benton et al., 1983)

Manual Dexterity/Laterality
Finger Tapping Test (Reitan & Davison, 1974)
Grooved Pegboard Test (Matthews & Klove, 1964)
Harris Test of Lateral Dominance (Harris, 1947)
Left/Right Hemisphere Scales (LNNB)
Purdue Pegboard (Purdue Research, 1948)
Purdue Perceptual-Motor Survey (Roach & Kephart, 1966)
Strength of Grip (Reitan & Davison, 1974)

Academic Achievement
Diagnostic [reading] Screening Procedure (Boder, 1973)
Kaufman Test of Educational Achievement (Kaufman & Kaufman, 1985)
Peabody Individual Achievement Test (Dunn & Markwardt, 1970)

(continued)

TABLE 17

CONTINUED

Reading/Everyday Activities in Life (Lichtman, 1972)
Wide Range Achievement Test - Revised (Jastak & Wilkinson, 1984)
WJ-R: Tests of Academic Achievement (Woodcock & Johnson, 1989)

Personality/Adjustment
Brief Psychiatric Rating Scale (Overall & Gorham, 1962)
Children's Apperception Test (Bellak & Bellak, 1974)
Draw A Person Projective Technique (Machover, 1948)
Katz Adjustment Scale (Katz & Lyerly, 1963)
Portland Adaptability Inventory (Lezak, 1980)
Personality Inventory for Children (Wirt, Lachar, Klinedinst, & Seat, 1977)
Roberts Apperception Test (Roberts & McArthur, 1982)
Rorschach Technique (1945)

Perception
Bender Visual Motor Gestalt (Bender, 1974)
Benton Visual Retention Test (Benton, 1974)
Block Design subtest (Wechsler scales)
Developmental Test of Visual Motor Integration (Beery, 1967)
Facial Recognition (Benton et al., 1983)
Fingertip Symbol Writing Recognition (Reitan & Davison, 1974)
Hooper Visual Organization Test (Hooper, 1983)
Map Localization Test (Benton, Levin, & Van Allen, 1974)
Minnesota Percepto-Diagnostic Test (Fuller, 1982)
Pantomime Recognition (Varney & Benton, 1982)
Speech Sounds Perception Test (Reitan & Davison, 1974)
Tactile Form Perception Test (Benton et al., 1983)
Tactual Performance Test (Reitan & Davison, 1974)
Trail Making Test (Reitan & Davison, 1974)
Underlining Test (Rourke & Gates, 1980)

Behavior
AAMD Adaptive Behavior Scale (Lambert, Windmiller, Tharinger, & Cole, 1981)
Adaptive Behavior Inventory for Children (Mercer & Lewis, 1978)
Boyd Developmental Progress Scale (Boyd, 1974)
Child Behavior Checklist (Achenbach & Edelbrock, 1986)
Conners Parent Rating Scale (Conners, 1985)
Conners Teacher Rating Scale (Conners, 1985)
Devereux Child/Adolescent Rating Scale (Spivack & Spotts, 1966)
Revised Behavior Problem Checklist (Quay & Peterson, 1983)
Vineland Adaptive Behavior Scales (Sparrow, Balla, & Cicchetti, 1984)

(continued)

TABLE 17

CONTINUED

Neuropsychological Batteries/Manuals

Benton Tests: A Clinical Manual (Benton et al., 1983)

Halstead-Reitan Battery (HRB) (Reitan & Davison, 1974)

Halstead-Reitan Neuropsychological Test Battery for Children (Reitan & Davison, 1974)

Halstead-Reitan Test Battery: An Interpretive Guide (Jarvis & Barth, 1984)

Lafayette Clinic Repeatable Neuropsychological Test Battery (Lewis & Kupke, 1977)

Luria-Nebraska Neuropsychological Battery (LNNB) (Golden, Hammeke, & Purisch, 1980)

Luria-Nebraska Neuropsychological Battery - Form II (Golden, Purisch, & Hammeke, 1985)

Luria-Nebraska Neuropsychological Battery - Children's Revision (LNNB-C) (Golden, 1987)

Reitan-Indiana Neuropsychological Test Battery for Children (Reitan & Davison, 1974)

Wechsler Adult Intelligence Scale - Revised as a Neuropsychological Instrument (WAIS-R NI) (Kaplan, Fein, Morris, & Delis, 1991)

Wisconsin Neuropsychological Test Battery (Harley, Leuthold, Matthews, & Bergs, 1980)

Psychological Assessment

The psychological assessment of traumatically brain-injured individuals should include formal and informal data; comparisons of preinjury and postinjury cognitive, educational, personality, and behavioral functioning; and practical treatment recommendations (see Table 18 for format for organizing and reporting neuropsychological data). Many of the standards for test administration and interpretation will need to be modified for the THI client. The predictive validity and reliability of common instruments and the analysis of formal results can no longer be viewed from a traditional context. The unique dimensions of traumatic brain injury will warrant methodological and interpretive adjustments. For example, special consideration must be given to preinjury characteristics, reactive complications, neurological factors, and the ongoing process of recovery, as each of these variables will have a bearing upon the instruments chosen, the methods and modifications used in test administration, and the extent to which performances are considered valid and reliable.

Although the Wechsler Full Scale IQ, Verbal IQ, and Performance IQ are among the most sensitive of all psychological measures in

TABLE 18

PSYCHOLOGICAL EVALUATION FOLLOWING THI:
A FORMAT FOR ORGANIZING AND REPORTING

I. **IDENTIFYING DATA**

II. **REASON FOR REFERRAL**
- Purpose of assessment
- Type of injury
- Time since injury

III. **TESTS ADMINISTERED** (adaptations noted)

IV. **BACKGROUND DATA**
- Relevant developmental/educational history
- Preinjury status
  1. estimated preinjury intellectual/academic status
  2. age and grade of child at injury
  3. preinjury behavior
- Current status
  1. description of current educational program and related services
  2. notable cognitive, physical, personality, or behavioral changes/ problems since injury
  3. parent, teacher, child perceptions of injury and its effects

V. **BEHAVIORAL IMPRESSIONS**
- Degree of alertness, orientation, motivation, attention
- Performance characteristics
  1. problem-solving strategies
  2. test-taking attitude
  3. error patterns
  4. self-monitoring behavior
  5. ability to make conceptual shifts
  6. attitude toward failure; frustration tolerance
  7. degree of persistence; motivation; stamina
  8. dexterity; hand preference
  9. optimal performance characteristics, e.g., preference for verbal vs. visual input; need for structure or redirection; optimal response mode; task preferences
  10. adjustment to injury

VI. **TEST RESULTS**
- Intellectual status (contrast with previous test results and/or evidence of best premorbid performance)
  1. statistically significant changes in cognitive subskills
  2. relative strengths and weaknesses

(continued)

TABLE 18

CONTINUED

- Academic achievement
  1. standard score comparisons
  2. compare with preinjury scores
  3. specific strengths and weaknesses
- Communication skills
  1. language abilities (reading, writing, listening, talking)
  2. articulation; intelligibility; pragmatics
- Motor functions
  1. hand preference (pre- and postinjury)
  2. fine and gross motor coordination (adequate or impaired)
- Perception (visual, auditory, tactile)
- Memory processes
  1. short-term/long-term
  2. verbal/nonverbal
  3. episodic/semantic
  4. visual/auditory
- Emotional and personality functioning

VII. **SUMMARY AND RECOMMENDATIONS**
- Overall impression of strengths and weaknesses in relation to:
  1. preinjury status
  2. current educational placement
  3. vocational goals
- Compensatory strategies
  1. strategies that optimize performance
  2. strategies that interfere with performance
  3. behavioral recommendations for school and home
  4. recommendations for classroom instruction
- Specific treatment recommendations
  1. retraining vs. compensation
  2. additional testing, referrals
  3. ancillary services
  4. projected date for reevaluation

VIII. **DATA SUMMARY SHEET**

Note. From "The Role of Assessment Following Traumatic Brain Injury" by V. Begali (in press). In R. C. Savage & G. F. Wolcott (Eds.), *Educational Programming for Children and Adults with Acquired Brain Injuries.* San Diego: College-Hill Press. Reprinted by permission with adaptations.

reflecting brain damage (Klonoff & Low, 1974; Lezak, 1983), the absence of a deficit-patterned profile (e.g., markedly inferior visuospatial skills, extreme intersubtest scatter, significant verbal-performance disrepancies [Chadwick & Rutter, 1983]) is not sufficient to conclude an absence of or recovery from neurological deficit (Boll, 1982; Lezak, 1983; Symonds, 1940). This fundamental tenet is borne out in follow-up studies of THI children and adolescents who regain essentially normal WISC-R profiles despite persistent memory, cognitive-processing, object-naming, and visuospatial deficits' which impinge upon their academic performance (Baxter et al., 1985; Chadwick, Rutter, Shaffer, & Shrout, 1981; Goldstein & Levin, 1985; Richardson, 1963). Despite its general sensitivity, few would dispute that the use of a Wechsler intelligence scale alone to infer the presence or absence of impairment is insufficient (Anastasi, 1982; Baxter et al., 1985, Boll & Barth, 1981; Lezak, 1983).

Intellectual measures have long been used to detect cognitive deterioration in cases of suspected neuropathology (Chelune, Ferguson, & Moehle, 1986). Although intellectual functioning as measured by the Wechsler scales appears to co-vary with the organic integrity of the brain, its ability to accurately reflect a loss of function is severely limited without the benefits of premorbid data for purposes of comparison (Leli & Filskov, 1979). The most direct method of detecting a loss of intellectual function following THI is to compare preaccident scores with postinjury scores. In most cases, however, premorbid intellectual and psychological data on THI students who had been making average or better-than-average academic progress prior to the injury are rarely available. Hence, former functioning must be estimated on the basis of educational and developmental history, teacher summaries, premorbid academic status (Richardson, 1963; Leli & Filskov, 1979; Matarazzo, 1972; Wilson, Rosenbaum, & Brown, 1979), or retrospective administration of behavior and personality surveys to the child's parents and former teachers. Because certain Wechsler subtest scores are less susceptible to the effects of brain injury (viz., Information, Vocabulary, Object Assembly, Picture Completion), they, too, can be used as rough indexes of former intellectual functioning (Prigatano, Pepping, & Klonoff, 1986; Wechsler, 1944). Conversely, the Wechsler subtests most sensitive to the effects of THI are Digit Symbol [Coding] and Block Design (Prigatano et al., 1986). Impaired performances on Digit Symbol or Coding subtests generally indicate psychomotor slowing, slowed information processing, and/or impaired learning.

Poor performance on Block Design may reflect impaired planning and organizational abilities, a visual-spatial disorder, or possible frontal lobe dysfunction (Luria & Tsvetkova, 1964).

For the vast majority of individuals (nearly all right-handers and approximately two-thirds of left-handed individuals [Reynolds, 1981]), the left cerebral hemisphere mediates linguistic, serial, and analytic functions; holistic and spatial tasks are primarily mediated by the right hemisphere (Chelune et al., 1986; Gazzangia, 1970; Luria, 1966; Sattler, 1982; Segalowitz & Gruber, 1977).

Lower Verbal and Performance IQs have been shown to correspond with lesions to the left and right hemispheres, respectively (Bornstein & Matarazzo, 1982; Lehr, 1990b; Luria, 1966). Woods (1980) determined that children who sustained unilateral brain damage prior to age 1 showed depressed Verbal and Performance IQs regardless of the side of damage. Those who sustained left-sided lesions later in childhood (mean age = 6 years) showed depressed Verbal and Performance IQs, although Reitan (1955) found PIQs to have been relatively less affected by left-sided lesions. Right-sided lesions, according to Woods, result in lower PIQs. Evidence also suggests that males may be more susceptible to the effects of Verbal and Performance IQ discrepancies due to unilateral lesions, whereas females are more likely to show a lowering of both verbal and performance scores irrespective of lesion laterality (Bornstein & Matarazzo, 1982; McGlone, 1978). The pattern of left (verbal) and right (performance) deficit is less distinct in individuals than it is for groups. For this reason, individual differences should be interpreted in light of other influential variables such as age, sex, premorbid status, educational background, handedness, time since injury, and degree of damage (Bornstein & Matarazzo, 1982; Chelune et al., 1986; Lezak, 1983; Rourke et al., 1983). It has been determined that Verbal IQ scores tend to recover within 6 to 12 months of the injury, whereas Performance IQs have been shown to take at least three times as long to recover (Becker, 1975; Chadwick, Rutter, Shaffer, & Shrout, 1981; Mandleburg & Brooks, 1975).

Educational Evaluation

When interpreting achievement test scores earned after a traumatic brain injury, the same cautions apply. Test results must be viewed in a context different from those of other students. Postinjury achievement scores simply reflect a student's ability to perform the specific tasks required at a point in time; they do not offer predictions of future academic performance (Cohen et al., 1985), nor do they confirm the complete return of academic functions. Achievement test results following THI become measures of long-term memory for well-learned material and do not necessarily represent a return of former scholastic status (Baxter et al., 1985). "Age" or "grade appropriate" scores are not proof that precursor skills remain intact, nor are they verification that continued achievement will occur in an orderly fashion. The comprehensive assessment of THI children and adolescents is a complex process. Because many functions are subject to disruption, many samples of behavior must be taken (Golden et al., 1980; Golden et al., 1983; Lezak, 1983).

Formal achievement test results can provide estimates of premorbid knowledge and learned engrams because well-learned skills are more resistant to the effects of THI (Golden, 1979; Rourke et al., 1983). A comparison of errors across tests can help pinpoint disturbed functions and damaged pathways. For example, by comparing mathematical performances from several different tests, one can parse out whether student difficulties are due to spatial problems, symbolic or numerical processing problems, or to a complete loss of memory for basic operations (Lezak, 1983).

Neurological and Neuropsychological Evaluation

Students reentering the public school system following a program of rehabilitation are likely to have undergone a neurological and neuropsychological assessment. A neurological examination includes information about the intactness of "lower level" functions such as those of the motor system and reflexes (Sattler, 1982; Tabaddor, 1982). The strength, efficiency, reactivity, and appropriateness of patient responses to motor commands, discrete stimulation of neural subsystems, and muscle groups are examined (Lezak, 1983). The neurologist generally assesses level of consciousness (using the Glasgow Coma Scale) by quantifying eye, motor, and verbal responses (Jennett & Teasdale, 1981). The position, movement, shape, and size of the eyes, and the reaction of the pupils to light, rotation, and flexion of the head are evaluated and inferences are drawn regarding cerebral intactness (Tabaddor, 1982).

The neuropsychologist, on the other hand, examines higher level cognitive processes such as intelligence, memory, and language (Golden, 1979; Incagnoli, Goldstein, & Golden, 1986; Lezak, 1983). Depending upon his or her training and orientation, the neuropsychologist may elect to offer added insights about personality and daily functioning, suggestions for intervention, and/or a prognosis for recovery.

Central to the rapid growth of clinical neuropsychology has been the success of neuropsychological testing procedures in detecting and localizing the presence of brain dysfunction (Caplan, 1982; Chelune et al., 1986). For THI persons, neuropsychological assessment offers a means by which individual strengths and weaknesses can be identified, degree of deficit and lesion site approximated, and program goals developed (Caplan, 1982; Rourke et al., 1983). With the routine use of computed tomography, positron emission tomography, and the impressive capabilities of magnetic resonance imaging to detect lesion sites, the field of neuropsychology is beginning to shift its emphasis from localization per se to the practical implications of brain damage upon daily functioning, prognosis, and educational and vocational goals (Incagnoli et al., 1986).

Neuropsychological measures differ from psychological tests in their focus and ability to detect changes in brain functioning (Goldstein, 1984). A range of neuropsychological, psychological, and special ability tests are typically used in neuropsychological evaluations. Lehr (1990b) contends that the principal difference between psychological and neuropsychological evaluations lies, not in the tests per se, but in the ways in which performance data are analyzed and put to use. Therefore, the distinction rests with the knowledge base (training) of the professional and the extent to which brain functioning is understood and its implications considered and applied. The tests administered for neuropsychological investigations are analyzed according to fundamental neuropsychological tenets. The data are typically organized to permit inferential analysis on the basis of level of performance, patterns of performance, pathognomonic signs, and a comparison of left- and right-sided efficiency (Boll, 1978; Reitan, 1968; Sattler, 1982; Selz, 1981). These inferential methods are described as follows:

1. *Level of Performance:* Standardized scores are compared to normative samples, criterion group, or an absolute standard of expectation. Cut-off points distinguish brain-damaged from non-brain-damaged persons.
2. *Patterns of Performance:* Relationships within a subgroup of tests or subtests are analyzed to ascertain strength or deficit patterns in an effort to infer lesion site and probable outcome.
3. *Pathognomonic Signs:* The presence of "soft" signs of dysfunction (e.g., rotation, constriction, perseveration, spatial neglect) and neurological "hard" signs (e.g. reflex abnormalities, asymmetrical and abnormal motor reflexes, absence of pupillary light reflex) are interpreted within the context of the complete evaluation to determine their significance.
4. *Comparison of Performance:* Sensory and motor efficiency of right and left body sides are compared and used to make inferences about the lateralization of damage and integrity of the hemispheres.

There is no simple one-to-one correspondence between discernible brain lesions and specific sensory, motor, or mental symptoms (Smith, 1975). The clinical assessment of brain–behavior relationships is a correlative and inferential process (Tarter & Edwards, 1986). Because neuropsychological tests are recognized for their sensitivity to changes in the condition of the brain, individual neuropsychological tests and neuropsychological reasoning should be used to augment standard psychological assessments (Goldstein, 1984), just as neuropsychological batteries are typically augmented by psychological, educational, and special ability tests and their respective rationales (Goldstein, 1986).

Neuropsychological assessments are generally conducted by means of a fixed or flexible battery of normed and standardized tests. In essence, battery approaches to neuropsychological assessment support the notion that performance is best measured via standardized test procedures and best interpreted against normed references. Two of the more popular fixed batteries most often used with children and adolescents have their roots in the early investigations of Ward Halstead and Alexander Luria. Although a number of other multifunctional batteries exist, only the child and adult versions of the Halstead-Reitan and Luria-Nebraska batteries are described in the following sections.

Comparatively, the flexible battery approach to neuropsychological assessment is more client-oriented and domain-specific. A variety of individual psychological, neuropsychological, and special ability tests are used to provide discrete and standardized measures of susceptible neurobehavioral functions with particular emphasis upon examination of areas of suspected dysfunction.

Kaplan (1988) advocates a *process-oriented approach* to neuropsychological assessment and interpretation whereby the client's behavior en route to a solution serves as the focus of investigative energies. Less emphasis is placed upon binary scoring and global results and greater emphasis is placed upon the assessment of optimal performance. The qualitative aspects of behavior are, however, quantified and subjected to statistical analyses and the testing of limits is operationally defined and repeatable. The process approach permits greater sensitivity to individual client variables, such as age, sex, handedness, family history, premorbid ability, etiology, and site of lesion. The Wechsler Adult Intelligence Scale - Revised (WAIS-R), a standard psychometric measure of cognitive functioning in older adolescents and adults, has recently been refashioned into a neuropsychological instrument (WAIS-R NI) (Kaplan, Fein, Morris, & Delis, 1991). This new instrument clearly embodies the philosophical and technical aspects of a process-oriented approach to neuropsychological assessment. A similar expansion of the WISC-III as a neuropsychological instrument is anticipated (E. Kaplan, personal communication, 1992).

Halstead-Reitan Batteries and Allied Procedures

In its current form, the Halstead-Reitan Battery (HRB) (age 15 and above) consists of five tests (Category Test, Tactual Performance Test [TPT], Speech-Sounds Perception Test, Finger Tapping Test, Seashore Rhythm Test). The battery is generally supplemented by "allied procedures," namely the appropriate Wechsler intelligence scale, an aphasia examination, a sensory-perceptual examination, the Trail Making Test, a measure of bilateral grip strength, and a measure of academic achievement and personality (Barth & Macciocchi, 1985). Several tests were either modified or eliminated from the HRB to comprise the intermediate and young children's versions: the *Halstead-Reitan Neuropsychological Test Battery for Children* (9-14 years) and the *Reitan-Indiana Neuropsychological Test Battery for Children*

(5-8 years). A description of the subtests included in these batteries can be found in Table 19.

The Halstead-Reitan batteries are essentially multifunctional laboratory approaches to neuropsychological assessment (Goldstein, 1986). The batteries are generally administered by specially trained technicians. A neuropsychologist conducts an interview and/or administers specialized testing procedures, and writes the report (Sattler, 1982). A battery may take up to 6 or more hours to administer. Few school psychologists have either the time to administer the Halstead-Reitan batteries or comprehensive training in their use; consequently, the Halstead-Reitan batteries are not considered a practical choice for the educational setting (Hartlage & Reynolds, 1981). Nevertheless, it is important to be familiar with the tests and bases for interpretation.

In order to assess the degree of brain dysfunction, the individual subtest scores on the HRB are used to formulate an "Impairment Index" (Russell, 1984). Over the years, the tests selected to make up the Impairment Index have changed on the basis of reliability and validity studies. At present, a summary value reflecting degree of dysfunction is calculated from the scores earned on the Category Test, Speech-Sounds Perception, Seashore Rhythm, and the three scores derived from the TPT. Impairment ratings can range from 0.0 to 1.0. An Impairment Index of 0.0 to 0.3 is indicative of normal functioning to mild cognitive impairment; 0.3 to 0.6 suggests mild to moderate dysfunction; 0.6 to 0.8, moderate to severe; and 0.8 to 1.0 indicates severe dysfunction (Barth & Macciocchi, 1985). Russell, Neuringer, and Goldstein (RNG) (1970) attempted to refine the Impairment Index to make it possible to reflect the degree of impairment with greater precision. Their revisions eventually led to the development of a computer program capable of analyzing and interpreting results on a 6-point scale (0-5) according to established norms; an average RNG rating of 4 or more is indicative of severe impairment (Russell, 1984).

The Halstead-Reitan batteries provide information of particular value in rehabilitative settings (Goldstein & Ruthven, 1983; Heaton & Pendleton, 1981; Heaton, Grant, Anthony, & Lehman, 1981). Individual programs of rehabilitation can be developed from an analysis of functioning patterns (Goldstein & Ruthven, 1983). Because the batteries are sensitive to changes in brain functioning, they are useful indices of progress over time.

TABLE 19

DESCRIPTION OF THE HALSTEAD-REITAN BATTERY (HRB),
THE HALSTEAD-REITAN NEUROPSYCHOLOGICAL TEST BATTERY FOR
CHILDREN (HNBC), AND THE REITAN-INDIANA NEUROPSYCHOLOGICAL
TEST BATTERY FOR CHILDREN (RINBC)

Test	Battery	Cognitive Functions Assessed
Seashore Rhythm Test	HRB, HNBC	Alertness, sustained attention, auditory perception, sequencing
Speech-Sounds Perception Test	HRB, HNBC	Attention, concentration, auditory perception, visual integration, judgment
Trail Making Test (Parts A & B)	HRB, HNBC	Flexibility, sequencing, scanning ability, symbolic appreciation
Sensory Perception	HRB, HNBC, RINBC	Sensory perception, attention
Strength of Grip	HRB, HNBC, RINBC	Motor strength of upper extremities
Lateral Dominance	HRB, HNBC, RINBC	Left-right preference
Category Test	HRB, HNBC, RINBC	Concept formation, intelligence, problem solving, new learning, flexibility
Tactual Performance Test	HRB, HNBC, RINBC	Somatosensory and sensorimotor ability, organization, problem solving
Finger Tapping Test	HRB, HNBC, RINBC	Fine motor speed
Aphasia Screening Test	HRB, HNBC, RINBC	Expressive and receptive language, spatial abilities, reading, writing
Matching Pictures Test	RINBC (opt.)	Perceptual recognition, attention
Individual Performance Tests	RINBC (opt.)	Visual perception, visual-motor ability
Marching Test	RINBC (opt.)	Gross motor control
Progressive Figures Test	RINBC (opt.)	Flexibility, abstraction, attention
Color Form Test	RINBC (opt.)	Flexibility, abstraction, language comprehension
Target Test	RINBC (opt.)	Memory for figures, attention, concentration, sequencing

Note. Appropriate allied procedures also administered (Wechsler Intelligence Scale, achievement test, special ability tests, personality inventory, etc.)

117

Luria-Nebraska Neuropsychological Battery (LNNB)

The LNNB (Golden, Hammeke & Purisch, 1980) is newer and therefore not as well established as the HRB. The LNNB (Form I, 1980, 1983) consists of 269 items which the authors contend represent approximately 700 procedures. The battery includes 11 ability scales, 2 sensorimotor scales, a pathognomonic scale, and localization and factor scales. Table 20 provides a description of the LNNB scales. The children's version of the LNNB consists of 149 items and includes the same clinical scales. The only distinction between the LNNB (12 years–adult) and the LNNB-C (8–12 years) is the exclusion of items that measure higher cognitive functions (viz., prefrontal skills) from the children's scale. Prior to age 12, few children are capable of sophisticated prefrontal processing (Golden, 1981b).

Golden and his associates developed the LNNB in an attempt to standardize Luria's (1966) clinical methods of evaluating brain-damaged patients. Behavioral observation, interviews, and other supplemental data are usually combined with the LNNB as they are with the HRB. Administration takes between 2-3 hours. The price of the LNNB is comparatively low (between $300 and $400) and its materials are portable.

Each scale attempts to measure the intactness of respective primary, secondary, and tertiary functions (Luria, 1966). Subscale scores are totaled and converted to T scores. A classification of dysfunction is determined by comparing actual performance on the scales with the performance expected of a person with the same age and level of education. A regression equation is used to predict a mean T score or baseline of performance. Subscale T scores above the critical level are considered abnormal (Golden & Maruish, 1986). The formula for critical level is:

$$68.8 + (.213 \times age) - (1.47 \times ed)$$

Age refers to chronological age in years except for individuals between 13 and 24 years. For 13 to 24 year olds, the age 25 years is used. Education (*ed*) refers to years in school. Brain damage is indicated when 3 or more of the scores from the 11 ability scales and the pathognomonic scale exceed the critical level. Profiles showing elevations on only those subtests sensitive to educational deficits (Reading, Writing, Arithmetic, Expressive Speech) should be

118

TABLE 20

DESCRIPTION OF THE LURIA-NEBRASKA NEUROPSYCHOLOGICAL
BATTERY - CHILDREN'S REVISION (LNNB-C) AND THE LURIA-NEBRASKA
NEUROPSYCHOLOGICAL BATTERY (LNNB)

Scale	Cognitive Functions Assessed
Motor	Bilateral motor speed, coordination, imitation, construction
Rhythm	Auditory discrimination, sequencing, memory, attention
Tactile	Finger and arm localization, two-point discrimination, shape discrimination, movement detection, attention
Visual	Visual recognition, visual memory, visual-spatial abilities
Receptive Speech	Receptive language, problem solving, flexibility, sequencing
Expressive Speech	Reading, expressive language, sentence repetition, memory, object naming, grammar
Writing	Spelling, copying, sequencing, memory, spontaneous writing
Reading	Sound synthesis, letter recognition, reading, writing
Arithmetic	Number recognition, number writing, simple and complex arithmetic operations
Memory	Short-term verbal and non-verbal memory, and paired-associate learning
Intelligence	General intelligence (comprehension, language, problem solving)
Pathognomonic	Consists of items drawn from 10 of the ability scales, "best indicator of brain integrity," highly sensitive to presence of brain dysfunction or overall impairment
Left hemisphere	Measures integrity of left-hemisphere sensorimotor strip (sensory and motor functions)
Right hemisphere	Measures integrity of right-hemisphere sensorimotor strip (sensory and motor functions)

Note. Adult battery subscales include additional items sensitive to formal operations. Spelling and Motor Writing are optional scales. Only Form II of the LNNB includes an Intermediate Memory Scale.

interpreted cautiously as such a profile may merely reflect the effects of poor schooling and not brain damage per se (Golden & Maruish, 1986).

The LNNB (Form II) (Golden, Purisch, & Hammeke, 1985) consists of 269 items which are essentially the same as those on the original form with only slight variations in content. Ten new items were added to form the Intermediate Memory Scale.

Comparing the HRB and LNNB

The literature generally regards both the HRB and LNNB as reliable and valid measures of neuropsychological functioning (Bennett, 1988; Golden, 1988; Golden & Maruish, 1986; Goldstein, 1986; McKay & Golden, 1979). Both are capable of lateralizing dysfunction and are sensitive to changes in brain function; they can discriminate brain-damaged from non-brain-damaged persons with approximately equal concurrent validity (Goldstein, 1986; Golden & Maruish, 1986). Both approaches are considered useful screening measures of language, memory, and motor skills (albeit to varying degrees) and both incorporate measures of general intelligence, visual-spatial abilities, attention, language, academic skills, perceptual and motor functions, and conceptual abilities (Golden & Maruish, 1986). Programs of rehabilitation can be derived from the data yielded by either the HRB or the LNNB (Goldstein, 1986). Goldstein compared the HRB and LNNB in an objective and well-presented overview. The highlights of his comparison which further distinguish these two popular batteries are summarized in Table 21.

Case Illustration. To provide the reader with a better idea of the neuropsychological changes that can follow THI, a case description and accompanying psychometric data follow.

A.R. (7 years old) sustained a severe closed head injury when struck by a car while crossing the street. She was a student in first grade and had been making average progress, although her behavior was somewhat impulsive and difficult to manage. Her initial Glasgow Coma Scale score was 8. She remained comatose for 7 days. Early CT scans (nonenhanced) revealed right frontal lobe damage and intracranial hemorrhage. She showed major left-sided hemiplegia and mild right hemiparesis. Her EEG was unremarkable for seizure activity, although phenobarbital was prescribed for 1 year as a preventative measure. After 3 weeks of pediatric intensive care, she was transferred to a child's rehabilitation center where she remained for 2 months. A.R. received daily individualized education, psychological services, and physical, occupational, speech, and recreational therapy. Her

TABLE 21

A COMPARISON OF THE HALSTEAD-REITAN BATTERY (HRB) AND THE
LURIA-NEBRASKA NEUROPSYCHOLOGICAL BATTERY (LNNB)

HRB	LNNB
1. Began as an extension of Halstead's theory of biological intelligence	1. Began as an extension of Luria's functional systems theory of brain organization
2. Published in 1947, better established and well researched	2. First published in 1979, reflects advantages of modern technology (e.g., the use of CT scans in validation studies)
3. Better at assessing nonverbal abilities in individuals with receptive language deficits	3. Better at identifying dysfunction in individuals with focal lesions (e.g., stroke, tumor, open head injury)
4. Stresses complex problem-solving and nonverbal abilities	4. Emphasizes language, language-related skills, and formal memory
5. Assesses fewer but more complex functions	5. Assesses a large number of discrete skills
6. IQ is assessed via Wechsler scale	6. IQ is estimated
7. Results are predictive of functional capability	7. Specific functional correlations are easy to generate from results
8. Requires permanent testing site, i.e., small office or laboratory	8. Portable materials, less expensive

first neuropsychological evaluation was conducted approximately 1 month following her injury (see Table 22). She was cooperative during testing, although easily distracted and prone to fatigue. Several testing sessions were required to complete the assessment. A.R.'s speech was noticeably impaired; she spoke in a slow monotonic voice which was slurred and difficult to understand. Her fine motor skills were poorly coordinated; she was barely able to use her left (nondominant) hand. Her gait was slow and awkward due to significant left-sided residual weakness. Test results showed significant intellectual impairment, particularly with respect to visual-perceptual processing, visual-motor speed, and precision. Her ability to discriminate forms on the basis of tactile cues (stereognosis) was impaired for both hands. Her ability

TABLE 22

CASE STUDY: DATA SUMMARY

Sex: Female   *Age at Injury:* 7 years

Premorbid characteristics: Normal development, average academic abilities, impulsive, strong-willed, right lateral preference

Neurological Exam: Unconscious; major left-sided hemiplegia; mild right hemiparesis

   Glasgow Coma Scale Score: 8   *PTA:* 10 days

Diagnostic Tests:
   CT Scan (without contrast): Right frontal lobe damage; intracranial hemorrhage; edema; no ventricular enlargement

   EEG: Normal; phenobarbital prescribed as prophylactic (preventative treatment)

Status at 5 years post injury: Left hemiparesis, mild affective disorder, conduct problems, residual learning deficits, left-sided visual neglect, visual-memory deficits

	Time Since Injury	
1 month		5 years
	Age at Testing	
7 years		12 years

Raw or Scaled Scores (Standard Scores)	Mean = 100/SD = 15	(Normal Range 85-115)	
	INTELLIGENCE (WISC-R)		
Verbal Subtests			
11 (105)	Information	10	(100)
12 (110)	Similarities	16	(130) +
11 (105)	Arithmetic	11	(105)
7 (85)	Vocabulary	11	(105) +
— 6 (80)	Comprehension	13	(115) +
9 (95)	Digit Span	7	(85)
Performance Subtests			
8 (90)	Picture Completion	10	(100)
— 4 (70)	Picture Arrangement	11	(105) +
8 (90)	Block Design	10	(100)
— 5 (75)	Object Assembly	12	(110) +
— 1 (55)	Coding	8	(90) +
(96)	VIQ		(113) +
— (69)	PIQ		(101) +
— (81)	FSIQ		(108) +
(95)	Intelligence Subtest (LNNB)		(112) +

(continued)

122

TABLE 22

CONTINUED

Raw or Scaled Scores (Standard Scores)		Mean = 100/SD = 15		(Normal Range 85-115)	
		ATTENTION/CONCENTRATION			
—	(80)	Arith., D.S., Coding		(91)	
	(86)	Rhythm subtest (LNNB)		(97)	
		LANGUAGE			
	(96)	VIQ		(113)	+
7	(85)	Vocabulary	11	(105)	+
		MEMORY			
9	(95)	Digit Span	7	(85)	
11	(105)	Information	10	(100)	
	(101)	Memory subtest (LNNB)		(106)	
		NEW LEARNING			
—	(69)	PIQ		(101)	+
39	(cut off score > 51)	Category test	30		
		ABSTRACT REASONING			
12	(110)	Similarities	16	(130)	+
6	(80)	Comprehension	13	(115)	+
		MANUAL DEXTERITY/LATERALITY (Finger tapping)			
— 14	(<67)	Dominant hand	35	(90)	+
— 0		Nondominant hand	27	(76)	+
		(Writing speed)			
— 65 sec.		Dominant hand	7 sec.		+
— 0		Nondominant hand	16 sec.		+
		ACADEMIC ACHIEVEMENT			
	(104)	Reading Recognition (WRAT)		(111)	
—	(82)	Reading Comprehension (PIAT)		(100)	+
	(98)	Spelling (WRAT)		(102)	
	(101)	Mathematics (WRAT)		(107)	
		VISUAL PERCEPTION			
—	(78)	Visual-motor integration (VMI)		(96)	+
— 5	(75)	Object Assembly	12	(100)	+
8	(90)	Block design	10	(110)	+
	(105)	Visual subtest (LNNB)		(115)	

(continued)

TABLE 22

CONTINUED

Raw or Scaled Scores (Standard Scores)			Mean = 100/SD = 15	(Normal Range 85-115)		
			TACTILE FUNCTIONS (Tactual Form Perception Test)			
—	5	(X = 8, SD = 1)	Dominant hand	(X = 9, SD = 1)	(9)	+
—	0	(X = 8, SD = 2)	Nondominant hand	(X = 9, SD = 1)	(8)	+
			Tactile subtest (LNNB)		(99)	

Note. – Significantly impaired at one month post injury.
    + Significant improvement at five years post injury (based upon increments of at least 1 SD or 15 SS points).

to attend and concentrate was markedly impaired, as was her comprehension for verbal and written material.

Upon reassessment at 5 years post injury, statistically significant improvements were noted on tests of abstract reasoning, judgment, word knowledge, and comprehension. She also showed significant improvement on a number of visual-perceptual, visual-motor, and dexterity tasks. Her Performance IQ "rose" 32 points, whereas her Verbal IQ, which was presumably less affected, "rose" 17 points. Mild word-retrieval difficulties, paraphasic errors, left-sided visual neglect, decreased sensory awareness, and poor visual-memory skills persisted. Socially, A.R. was experiencing interpersonal problems with her peers. By the time of her 5-year follow-up, she had been suspended twice for aggressive behavior and a "disrespectful attitude." Evidence of mild to moderate depression was clinically assessed and believed to be due to the interaction of social isolation, poor peer relationships, an awareness of her deficits, and familial pressures.

Re-evaluation

School psychologists are encouraged to request the psychological, neurological, neuropsychological, and medical records of the THI clients school systems intend to serve. It is wise to solicit pragmatic interpretations of formal findings and recommendations for further treatment prior to student re-entry. Medical, rehabilitative, and psychometric data provide the necessary background and baseline for treatment and subsequent school-based evaluations.

Given that recovery from head injury can continue for years (Beaumont, 1983; Boll, 1983; Chadwick, Rutter, Shaffer, & Shrout, 1981; Lezak, 1983; Richardson, 1963; Rimel, Giordani, Barth, Boll, & Jane, 1981; Ylvisaker, 1985), the results of posttrauma assessments need to be interpreted with the recognition that further recovery is always possible. The results of an assessment conducted at 5 or even 10 months post injury are less reliable and much more likely to change than those conducted at 5 years post injury (Chadwick, Rutter, Shaffer, & Shrout, 1981; Rimel et al., 1981). Moreover, the test scores of traumatically head-injured children and adolescents are likely to fluctuate considerably during the first few years after the injury (Rourke et al., 1983). Unless an individual's deficits are so severe, it is unwise to make binding judgments about mental status until several years have passed (Lezak, 1983).

Frequent reevaluation of head-injured students is recommended (Levin et al., 1983; Sattler, 1982). Barth and Macciocchi (1985) suggest that reassessment be conducted at regular (3-6 month) intervals over the first several years. Serial assessments may be spaced further apart once general performance begins to plateau (Levin & Goldstein, 1989). All follow-up assessments should take into account the effects of practice, as shorter intervals and repeated use of the same instrument can produce inflated test scores. Both alternative tests and test forms supplemented by criterion-based data should be used when assessment intervals are less than one year (Sattler, 1988). Improved retest scores may be an indication of spontaneous recovery, intervention efforts, test error, or test familiarity. As a general rule, a difference of one standard error of measurement corroborated by other formal and informal data is indicative of statistical significance, i.e., meaningful change, not simply due to chance (Lezak, 1987; Sattler, 1988). On initial postinjury testing, THI children and adolescents are less likely to benefit from practice effects on attention and memory tasks, in particular, than their noninjured counterparts (Brooks, 1987). On subsequent testing, however, THI students will often show greater practice effects than noninjured students (Lehr, 1990b). Informal assessment is the recommended companion to standardized procedures. Routine samples of

125

criterion- or curriculum-based performance form the practical basis for instructional efforts and offset the inherent limitations of formal measures (Anastasi, 1982).

Their characteristic potential for rapid and variable change makes THI children and adolescents a unique population; no other category of exceptional learners can claim potential for a "gain" of as many as 30 IQ points within one year (Chadwick, Rutter, Shaffer, & Shrout, 1981). Significant and variable changes are common within head-injured persons. These changes may well justify significant programmatic and instructional revisions. In order to maximize the period of recovery immediately following the injury and beyond, a systematic and careful plan for education and rehabilitation must be implemented (Rutter, 1981). Periodic reassessment makes it possible to monitor progress, revise instructional objectives, and correct program deficiencies. The reassessment process should aim to:

1. Establish a baseline performance from which to measure progress over time.
2. Reexamine the student's special service needs.
3. Detect specific areas of dysfunction or problems in the performance of basic motor, academic, cognitive, and social/emotional functions.
4. Determine the success or failure of various treatments.
5. Modify instructional objectives, program, and placement on a timely basis.
6. Redirect and revitalize team efforts (Begali, in press).

10

TREATMENT RATIONALE AND STRATEGIES FOR THE EDUCATIONAL SETTING

Before attempting to implement specific treatment strategies, it is useful to develop a theoretical grounding and sense of direction. When determining methods of treatment, an assortment of variables need to be considered, namely, the age of the child, extent of injury, pattern of strengths and weaknesses, premorbid functioning, and stage of recovery. This chapter provides school and allied professionals with a conceptual grounding in treatment rationale and the principles of intervention following THI. A range of techniques that fall within the broad categories of cognitive rehabilitation, behavioral management, and psychological and psychiatric intervention are subsequently discussed. Table 23 identifies over 50 specialized cognitive, behavioral, and psychosocial interventions.

Conceptual Models of Remediation

The treatment of traumatically head-injured clients calls for a blend of special skills and varied strategies. When providing educational treatment to THI students it will be necessary to borrow from the principles of several relevant disciplines.

1. *Developmental psychology.* Traumatically brain-injured individuals tend to regain lost cognitive functions along a hierarchical sequence, that is, the reacquisition and stabilization of lower level processes generally precedes the reemergence of higher level functions (Hagen, 1981). Developmental milestones may be used to formulate goals of treatment during the early stages of recovery or as

TABLE 23

SELECTED COGNITIVE, BEHAVIORAL, AND PSYCHOSOCIAL
INTERVENTIONS FOLLOWING THI

Problem	Intervention	Study/Source
Cognitive		
Processing deficits	Compensatory training	Diller & Gordon, 1981
Processing deficits	Cognitive retraining	Ben-Yishay et al., 1982
Poor reasoning, judgment, and problem solving	Systematic practice and guidance	Richman & Gholson, 1978
Poor planning	Overt verbal self-regulation of behavior, faded to "inner" speech	Cicerone & Wood, 1987
General cognitive deficits	Video games	Lynch, 1982
Attention deficits	Stimulant medication	Evans & Gualtieri, 1987
Word finding disability	Verbal praise for improvement in the number of objects named per 60-sec interval	Ince, 1976
Learning deficits	Sensory integration therapy	Ayres, 1972
Learning deficits	Computer assisted learning	Lynch, 1986, 1989
Aphasia	Melodic intonation therapy; stimulation of nondominant hemisphere	Albert, Sparks, & Helm, 1973
Aphasia	Symbolic artificial language training	Glass, Gazzangia, & Premack, 1973
Aphasia	Visual communication	Gardner, Zurif, Berry, & Baker, 1976
Poor memory	Memory therapy group	Wilson & Moffat, 1984
Poor memory	Reality Orientation Therapy (ROT)	Wilson & Moffat, 1984; Sohlberg & Mateer, 1989
Poor memory	Computer assisted learning	Kurlycheck & Glang, 1984
Poor memory	Mnemonic devices, self-instruction, guided inquiry, visual imagery	Rusch, Grunert, Erdmann, & Lynch, 1980

(continued)

TABLE 23

CONTINUED

Problem	Intervention	Study/Source
Poor memory	Visual imagery	Deelman, Berg, & Koning-Haanstra, 1990; Lewinsohn, Danaher, & Kikel, 1977
Poor memory	Memory book	Sohlberg & Mateer, 1989
Poor memory	Oral rehearsal; system for asking key questions; visual imagery	Glasgow, Zeiss, Barrera, & Lewinsohn, 1977
Poor memory	Chaining words through bizarre imagery	Crovitz, Harvey, & Horn, 1979
Visual perceptual deficits	Microcomputers and software	Bracy, 1985; Lynch, 1989
Repetitive speech	Response cost, cognitive overlearning	Alderman & Burgess, 1990
Behavioral		
Aggression	Regime of time-out, token reinforcement, and social skills training	Wood, 1987
Aggression	Anticonvulsant medication plus behavioral management	Cassidy, 1990; Wood, 1987
Belligerent and disruptive behavior	Ignore disruptions; reinforce positive behavior with attention, physical contact, active listening	Hollon, 1973
Belligerent and disruptive behavior	Differential reinforcement of other (incompatible) behavior	Lovell, 1987
Belligerent and disruptive behavior	Temporary time-out, removal of potential for reinforcement	Wood, 1987
Tantrums; avoidance of physical therapy	Time-out; token reinforcement for task compliance exchanged by day for tangible rewards, faded to praise	Sand, Trieschman, Fordyce, & Fowler, 1970
Poor behavior controls	Cognitive Behavior Modification (CBM)	Meichenbaum, 1977

(continued)

129

TABLE 23

CONTINUED

Problem	Intervention	Study/Source
Impulsivity	Self-talk; self-instruction	Meichenbaum & Goodman, 1971; Sohlberg & Mateer, 1989
Poor attention	Tokens for attending behavior delivered at increasing intervals	Wood, 1987
Poor attention	Stimulant medication	Evans & Gualtieri, 1987
Lack of motivation	Social attention for the maintenance or increase of productive on-task behavior; bar graph of progress	Taylor & Persons, 1970
Poor participation	Admittance to desired activity contingent upon participation in undesired activity	Ince, 1969
Poor participation	Points for responding within specified time limit	Wood, 1987
Poor self-initiation	Response-cost/reinforcement	Nelson, Finch, & Hooke, 1975
Tactile defensiveness	Desensitization plus time-out	Wood, 1987
Inappropriate sexual behavior	Simultaneous treatment of sexual and aggressive behavior using time-out and response cost	Wood, 1987
Psychosocial		
Uncooperative, negativistic attitude	Utilization of negative behavior (paradoxic directive); require client to engage in the avoidant or targeted behavior	Kushner & Knox, 1973
Anger about injury	Play therapy	Schaefer & O'Connor, 1983
Lack of initiative	Assertiveness training	Salter, 1961
Habit disorders	Massed practice followed by positive punishment	Wood, 1987
Poor coping skills	Rational-Emotive Therapy	Ellis, 1975

(continued)

TABLE 23

CONTINUED

Problem	Intervention	Study/Source
Poor conversational skills	Interpersonal Process Recall	Helffenstein, 1981; Kagan, 1969
Inappropriate social behaviors	Videotaped interactions and critique	Helffenstein & Wechsler, 1982
Inappropriate social behaviors	Social competence training	Hopewell, Burke, Weslowski, & Zawlocki, 1990
Inappropriate social behaviors	Structured learning	Goldstein, Sprafkin, Gershaw, & Klein, 1980
Inappropriate social behaviors	Pragmatic skills training	Mateer & Ruff, 1990
Complaining	Attention withheld when complaining; attention provided for noncomplaining talk	Taylor & Persons, 1970
Absence of interpersonal gaze	Negative auditory feedback for gaze aversion	Diller, 1980
Depression, interpersonal conflict	Cognitive therapy, psychoanalytic theory, insight and introspection	Prigatano, 1991; Stern, 1985

broad markers of progress. Piaget's (1969) notions of assimilation and accommodation provide a basis for developing instructional objectives and treatment strategies. Cognitive growth becomes the balance between the organization of information in terms of what is currently known or remembered (assimilation) and the integration of new information and properties through constant reorganization or recovery (accommodation). Because head-injured youngsters frequently experience problems with memory and organization, it will be necessary to structure tasks from simple to complex (Adamovich, Henderson, & Auerbach, 1985). Both chronological and developmental age should be considered when developing goals for treatment (Szekeres et al., 1985).

2. *Neuropsychology.* Certain behaviors may be disrupted because of damage to particular areas of the brain. By identifying the breakdown of specific skills (functions), alternate intact skills (pathways) can be used to achieve the desired goal (Diller, 1980; Golden, 1981a; Luria, 1973; Rourke et al., 1983). For example, visual feedback can be substituted for kinesthetic feedback when retraining an individual with kinesthetic dysfunction to walk (Bolger, 1982). The length of strides can be guided by visual markers placed on the floor. Luria's theories of brain organization and function offer a conceptual reference for practitioners seeking explanations of cerebral dysfunction or the recovery process, and a rationale for remediation. Neuropsychological principles provide a sensitive basis and compatible framework for the assessment and retraining of brain-injured persons.

3. *Behavioral psychology.* Social awareness, initiative, judgment, and the cognitive integration required to translate environmental cues into adaptive responses are often impaired by THI. For these reasons, less complex and more systematic methods of rehabilitation are recommended. A structured environment that promotes practice and repetition, consistent and reasonable expectations, behavioral contingencies, and clear and responsive feedback eases undue reliance upon the very skills THI individuals so often lack (Gordon et al., 1985; Wood, 1990b). Although cognitive and information-processing capabilities are needed to understand the relationship between behavior and the environment, conditioning techniques can promote learning in the absence of cognitive insight and self-awareness without placing an unnecessary burden upon weakened cognitive functions (Wood, 1990b). By assessing the learning potential and capacity to modify behavior in response to systematically altered environmental contingencies, strategies for improving behavior can be derived (Ben-Yishay & Diller, 1983).Brain-injured individuals can be conditioned to profit from different degrees of cueing. Their behavior can be directed by providing continuous feedback and cues across tasks of increasing difficulty (Adamovich et al., 1985; Ben-Yishay & Diller, 1983; Szekeres et al., 1985). Behavioral approaches can help reshape necessary skills into a form that resembles the ideal, while specifying the sequence and conditions under which the target behavior should occur. Accordingly, rehabilitation efforts may be built upon directed

behavioral responses that are prompted by specific environmental cues, rewards, practice, and overlearning (Begali, 1987; Gordon et al., 1985).

4. *Special education.* Psychological processing theories that advocate "training the deficit" and "teaching through the preferred modality" (Johnson & Myklebust, 1967) have been applied to head-injured persons (Diller, 1976; Luria, 1963; Rourke et al., 1983). The multi-sensory approach (Fernald, 1943), sensory integration training (Ayres, 1972), and perceptual training (Wepman, 1968) have also found their way into treatment programs for head-injured youngsters and are applicable with individualized modification. Individualized program planning, regularly scheduled reevaluations of learning needs, and related services are likely components of an educational plan for head-injured persons. The current political move afoot to form a partnership between general and special education represents a process of reform that holds promise for traumatically brain-injured students. Innovative programs such as "adaptive learning," "individually guided education," and "team-assisted individualization" combine the best of contemporary initiatives (Wang et al., 1989). Such reform is intended to promote a reliance upon cooperative educational interventions that are aimed at accommodating the unique learning needs and abilities of individual students. Materials, procedures, and activities are selected with the specific needs and interests of each student in mind.

Approaches to Remediation

Philosophical differences and emphases distinguish the various approaches to neurological rehabilitation. Fundamentally, all remedial approaches are either direct or compensatory in nature. Whether it is best to attack neuropsychological deficiencies directly or to help compensate for their effects through internal or external strategies depends upon the age of the child, stage of recovery, type and degree of impairment, the child's ability to respond, and his or her degree of receptiveness (see Figure 11). A description of three treatment approaches follows.

1. *Direct retraining of underlying neuropsychological weakness.* This method of providing direct remediation for neuropsychological deficiencies is most appropriate for (a) children under 12 years of

FIGURE 11

REMEDIAL APPROACHES FOLLOWING TRAUMATIC BRAIN INJURY

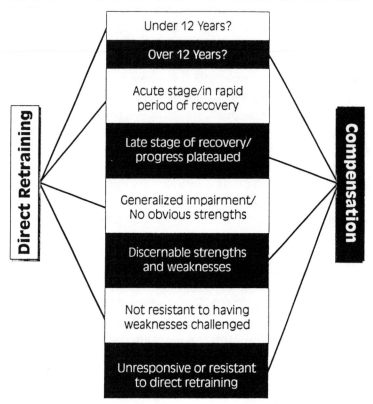

of age, because their brains have not yet reached maturity and, as such, are likely to undergo substantial cerebral reorganization; (b) children and adolescents during the acute stage of the injury and in a rapid period of recovery; (c) children and adolescents whose deficiencies respond to such treatment and who are not resistant to having their weaknesses challenged; and (d) those whose brain damage has produced a generalized derangement with little or no obvious sparing of function (i.e., strengths).

2. *Compensatory training/functional restoration.* Underlying the compensatory approach lies the premise that cognitive functioning cannot be improved by direct training alone (Haarbauer-Krupa, Henry, Szekeres, & Ylvisaker, 1985; Luria, 1963; Miller, 1984;

Szekeres et al., 1985). Compensatory training is recommended for (a) older children and adolescents who tend to deny their deficits and who resist direct retraining; (b) those whose strengths and weaknesses are specific and easily identified; (c) younger and older children whose neuropsychological deficiencies are resistant to direct remediation; and (d) those whose progress by alternate methods has plateaued (Luria, Naydin, Tsvetkova, & Vinarskaya, 1969; Miller, 1984; Rourke et al., 1983). The success of compensatory training depends upon the mobilization of residual skills (strengths) to achieve an otherwise unobtainable goal. For example, internal strategies such as self-instructional talk (Meichenbaum & Goodman, 1971), visual scanning (Avidan, 1977), auditory rehearsal (Wilson & Moffat, 1984), and gestures and sign language (Skelly, 1979), when intact, can be used to enhance or supplant deficit functions. External aids such as timers, alarm systems, log books, tape recorders, calculators, charts, graphs, mnemonics, large print books, and communication boards can also be used to compensate for unresponsive deficit functions.

3. *Process-specific training.* Sohlberg and Mateer (1989) advocate a process-specific approach whereby direct retraining and compensatory techniques are systematically integrated. Treatment efforts are aimed at the restoration of specific neurological functions through repetition and direct training. Compensatory strategies are accessed when restoration to a functional level is not possible. Unlike the aforementioned approaches to rehabilitation, the selective and systematic presentation of remedial tasks and progress measurement are emphasized in the process-specific approach. In order to facilitate the measurement of treatment efficacy, hierarchically organized treatment goals are data-based and generalization probes are used. Individual improvement is measured on the basis of increased vocational potential and independent living capabilities.

Principles of Intervention

Szekeres et al. (1985) identified seven principles that apply to intervention practices based upon their experiences with head-injured children and adolescents. Some modification has been made by this author.

Principle 1: Success resulting from planned compensation and appropriate expectations facilitates [student] progress while building a productive self-concept.

Principle 2: The systematic gradation of activities facilitates cognitive recovery and development by ensuring successful performance in a controlled and cumulative manner.

Principle 3: Habituation and generalization training are necessary for learning and carryover.

Principle 4: Student initiation, motivation, and goal selection facilitate recovery and are essential for effective and independent functioning.

Principle 5: Integration of treatment, recreational activities, and compensatory strategies among staff and family members promotes consistency and facilitates the student's orientation, learning, and generalization of learned skills.

Principle 6: Chronological and developmental age must be considered in treatment design to ensure appropriate and attainable objectives.

Principle 7: Individual and group treatment options provide specificity of intervention as well as reality-based training in social cognition.

Stage of Recovery

The stages of recovery outlined in chapter 5 illustrate the evolution of the recovery process following severe head trauma. Stage of recovery has little to do with time-since-injury, however, because individuals can plateau at "early" or "middle" stages and remain there indefinitely. Those falling within the Early Stage of Recovery (Levels I, II, III) will require regulated sensory and sensorimotor stimulation alternated by frequent and quiet rest periods, to facilitate arousal and adaptive responses to the environment (Wood, 1991). Those who fall within the Middle Stage of Recovery (Levels IV, V, VI) will require highly structured environmental adjustments and the systematic gradated retraining of cognitive functions (Szekeres et al., 1985). For example, a student may need to relearn organizational and attention skills or practical problem-solving strategies. Eventually, these individuals may be graduated to more demanding tasks that require greater degrees of attention, selectivity, discrimination, and filtering. As demands are increased, prompts, cues, and structure are systematically decreased (Diller, 1976). Direct functional retraining may also be required: Students may need to practice conversational skills, proper facial expression, or behavioral inhibition (Haarbauer-Krupa, Moser, Smith, Sullivan, & Szekeres, 1985).

The Late Stage of Recovery (Levels VII, VIII) calls for a focus on developing independence and adaptability within increasingly more normalized environments. During this stage too, students may need direct instruction on how to interact appropriately, communicate in a conventional way, abide by social codes, and remember details. Some deficits may require environmental adjustments (Rourke et al., 1983). For example, a reduced course load, collapsed school day, modified expectations, or the elimination of time limits may be necessary. Some THI students will require compensatory training for resistant difficulties.

Classroom Instruction and Cognitive Rehabilitation

The effects of traumatic brain injury vary from individual to individual and from brain to brain. No two injuries produce the same results. Premorbid diversity interacts with varying degrees and causes of trauma to produce variable outcomes. Goals, strategies, priorities, and services need to be adjusted according to the specific yet changing needs of the child with traumatic brain injury. Table 24 provides a hierarchy of broad-based objectives and general strategies according to cognitive functioning level (refer to Levels of Cognitive Functioning, Table 11). The objectives may be individualized by gradually increasing the rate, amount, and duration of stimulus input and requiring increasingly more complex methods of response (Hagen, 1981). The manner in which the strategies are implemented will vary according to degree of deficit, stage of recovery, age, and intact versus damaged functions. The table represents an integration of the works of Adamovich, Henderson, and Auerbach (1985), Smith and Ylvisaker (1985), Hagen (1981), Ylvisaker (1985), and the clinical experiences of this author. Particular attention has been paid to the Late Stage of Recovery because school personnel are most likely to be faced with the subtle and persistent symptoms of individuals who reenter at this level. Appendix A offers a list of educational resources and sources of supplemental computer software programs appropriate for THI students.

TABLE 24

GOALS AND STRATEGIES FOR PROMOTING RECOVERY BY
LEVEL OF COGNITIVE FUNCTION

EARLY STAGES OF RECOVERY

Level of Cognitive Functioning: **I, II**
(No Response; Generalized Response)

Goals:
1. Prevent sensory deprivation
2. Elicit responses to sensory stimuli
3. Increase frequency, rate, variety, and quality of responses

Strategies:
Provide regulated stimulation (15–30 minute intervals alternated with periods of quiet rest) by means of:
1. Colorful familiar objects (favorite toys, books, pictures)
2. Frequent verbal interaction
3. T.V. (used intermittently to prevent satiation)
4. Audio tapes of familiar voices and favorite music
5. Contact with various textures, temperatures, densities
6. Visual tracking exercises (vertical, horizontal, circular)
7. Auditory localization and auditory tracking exercises (recordings of familiar people, music)
8. Olfactory stimulation (varied natural and familiar odors, e.g., coffee beans, vanilla, spices)
9. Varied settings and body position changes
10. Simple sorting and matching activities (color, shape, size, sound to picture, word to picture)

Level of Cognitive Functioning: **III**
(Localized response)

Goals
1. Develop ability to attend
2. Develop ability to follow commands
3. Develop ability to use objects appropriately
4. Establish means of communication

Strategies
1. Involve in movement activities (e.g., gentle rocking, mat activities)
2. Provide tactile stimulation activities (different textures, densities, temperatures)
3. Develop simple matching skills (meaningful pictures, shapes, colors, words, sounds)
4. Involve in minimal self-care tasks (overlearned skills with prompting, e.g., hair brushing, use of wash cloth and eating utensils)
5. Utilize high-interest simple video games

(continued)

TABLE 24

CONTINUED

6. Engage in one-step commands with prompting (e.g., "squeeze my hand," "look at me," "close your eyes")
7. Continue olfactory and add gustatory stimulation
8. Encourage communication no matter how primitive (use gestures, pictureboard, simple yes/no system)
9. Provide orientation drills (e.g., name?, age?, day?, week?, year?)
10. Introduce simple choice-making opportunities

MIDDLE STAGES OF RECOVERY

Level of Cognitive Functioning: IV
(Confused-Agitated)

Goals:
1. Decrease intensity, duration, and frequency of agitation
2. Increase attention to environment
3. Prevent purposeless responses

Strategies:
1. Keep environment predictable
2. Increase human contact
3. Limit demands to simple one-step requests
4. Continue reality orientation therapy (e.g., setting, time, date, school, family)
5. Involve in sequencing activities (numerical ordering, size gradation activities, letter ordering to form familiar words)
6. Review prepositions. Use objects to redevelop concepts such as on, under, in, beside, over, etc.
7. Encourage participation in simple self-care tasks
8. Permit group interactions either as participant (when possible) or as observer

Level of Cognitive Functioning: V, VI
(Confused-Inappropriate, Confused-Appropriate)

Goals:
1. Decrease confusion and improve self-awareness
2. Develop attention and selective attention skills
3. Increase environmental interactions
4. Facilitate short-term memory skills through simple conversation, questioning, and restatement
5. Increase cognitive function by means of structure and repetition
6. Begin continence training (Level V)
7. Begin formal assessment (Level VI)

Strategies:
1. Call attention to relevant stimuli, minimize distractions

(continued)

TABLE 24

CONTINUED

2. Provide for redundancy, repetition, and practice
3. Utilize memory aids such as clocks, calendars, daily schedules, notebooks
4. Continue reality orientation training
5. Encourage emotional expression and discussion
6. Involve in graded visual-motor tasks, i.e., tracing, copying designs, discrimination, simple assembly, and visual closure exercises (e.g., supply missing letter or element)
7. Correct inaccurate verbal responses/misconceptions, etc.
8. Encourage repetition of words, phrases, and sentences. Increase rate, amount, duration, and complexity of stimuli
9. Conduct sequencing activities using numerals; letters ordered to form words; words to form sentences; multi-step commands
10. Develop simple association and categorization skills using real objects, then pictures, then words. Utilize different modes of input (visual, auditory) and require different forms of output (visual, motor, verbal)
11. Encourage group participation and socialization
12. Emphasize resumption of daily living skills
13. Involve in paper and pencil tasks
14. Introduce increasingly more difficult visual discrimination exercises (tones, shapes, sizes, words, sentences, embedded figures, etc.)
15. Pre-academics: simple calculation, reading recognition/comprehension, written language. Reestablish productive work habits
16. Provide for directed social interaction/cooperation exercises
17. Provide for drills on daily schedule, orientation, ordering, retention
18. Involve in simple cognitive software programs

LATE STAGES OF RECOVERY

Level of Cognitive Functioning: VII, VIII
(Automatic-Appropriate, Purposeful-Appropriate)

Goals:
1. Decrease dependence upon structure, increase responsibility
2. Reintroduce to community
3. Facilitate insight into his/her condition. Develop self-awareness
4. Develop sequential thought processing, organization, reasoning, and problem solving

Strategies:
1. Gradually reduce dependency upon structure and memory aids where possible
2. Increase demands for student responsibility, i.e., appointments, clean-up, assignments

(continued)

TABLE 24

CONTINUED

3. Develop practical problem-solving skills through discussion, role playing, videotaped simulation exercises
4. Discuss deficits and their implications. Brainstorm possible compensatory strategies
5. Enhance values clarification through discussion, small group activities, simulation exercises
6. Reinforce independence in personal care, daily routine
7. Refine social skills (simple courtesies, table manners, conversation, telephone use, dating, assertiveness)
8. Refine basic academic skills. Stress functional skills (e.g., filling out forms, job applications, money management)
9. Plan for prevocational and vocational training. Refer to local Department of Rehabilitative Services, DRS
10. Gradually develop community competence through supervised and semi-supervised practical experience

Additional Cognitive Retraining Treatments
(Adamovich, Henderson, & Auerbach, 1985; Ben-Yishay, 1980; Bracy, 1983; Schmidt & Lynch, 1983; Sohlberg & Mateer, 1989)
1. Retention, storage, retrieval, organization
   a. Visual (via paper-pencil tasks, manipulation, computer software, or practical activities)
      (1) discrimination and tracking exercises
      (2) visual reaction/responsiveness (video games)
      (3) gradated reading exercises
      (4) memory improvement (mnemonic strategies, e.g., chunking, visual imagery, rehearsal, categorization)
      (5) visual-motor training (drills to increase speed and precision)
   b. Auditory (via discussion, paper-pencil tasks, audio tapes, or computer software)
      (1) serial memory (words, then sentences)
      (2) comprehension exercises
      (3) long-term memory drills
2. Sequential thought, reasoning, problem solving (via paper-pencil tasks, discussion, video and audio tapes, computer software, practical experiences, role playing, counseling, video therapy)
   a. advanced analysis and categorization exercises
   b. hypothetical problem solving (what should you do if . . . ?)
   c. identification of similarities and differences in concrete then abstract entities
   d. interpretation of morals, proverbs, fables, idioms, riddles
   e. analogies (back is to front as down is to _____); verbal absurdities
   f. social skills training, video therapy, group discussion, simulation exercises
   g. grammatical proofing exercises
   h. recognition of potentially harmful situations and identification of precautions

(continued)

TABLE 24

CONTINUED

---

    i. organized decision making and practice for reality (values clarification exercises; hypothetical problem solving)

    j. review of basic skills and applied academics

    k. plan, execute, and self-evaluate independent community participation (What do you need to go shopping?; How will you get there?; How do you ask for a date?; If lost, how would you go about finding your way home?)

3. Insight, judgment, formulation of appropriate goals

    a. discuss effects of brain damage and current status

    b. group counseling (peer modeling, role playing, discussion, peer review)

    c. target specific cognitive, social, and vocational goals, formulate written plans of action

    d. plan strategies for accomplishment of short and long-term goals

    e. develop leisure time preferences

    f. sex education (sexual responsibility, contraception, health issues, values clarification, dating, marriage, children)

Academic Retraining

Intrasubtest analysis of student performance on tests of academic achievement, informal surveys, neuropsychological and psychological assessments, speech/language evaluations, preaccident academic history, and observations will provide the individualized criteria from which to develop instructional goals and treatment strategies. It is important to be mindful of the possibility that very basic concepts may be lost or disorganized in spite of a seemingly adequate psychometric profile. It is also possible for THI students to have retained a number of isolated skills at their preinjury level despite a range of seriously compromised areas of functioning (Rourke et al., 1983). As a rule, previously weak areas of academic functioning tend to become weaker as a result of brain trauma. THI will not improve former academic capability (Rosen & Gerring, 1986).

Due to the paucity of research on prescriptive instructional metholodogy for THI students (Miller, 1984) and the inherent heterogeneity of this group of learners, practitioners are left to assume that sound teaching practices adapted to the learner and delivered with an appreciation for the possible sequelae of head injury have the same chance for success as they do when applied knowingly to other disabled learners (Cruikshank, Bentzen, Ratzeburg, & Tannhauser, 1961; Heward & Orlanksy, 1980). Task analysis, systematic and structured programs, individualized plans, and compensatory training are sound and recommended teaching practices (Hallahan et al., 1983) and are appropriate for THI youngsters (Cohen et al., 1985). Instructional programs for the THI student should stimulate a variety of processing modes, although direct instruction is best presented through the student's single most intact sensory modality in order to minimize distraction (Cohen et al., 1985; Hagen, 1981). The practice of simultaneous sensory "bombardment" is inappropriate for most THI youngsters.

Few THI-specific teaching techniques are recognized in the literature, although some studies on acquired dyslexia and acquired dyscalculia have surfaced (Miller, 1984). During the initial post-traumatic stages of reading recovery, Gheorghita (1981) suggests that material be presented in a vertical rather than horizontal format. In this way, instruction progresses from vertically aligned (column fashion) letters ordered to form words, to a column of syllables that form a word, to words that form sentences. Once visual-spatial and visual-scanning skills improve, a gradual transition to horizontal presentation is made. Other studies of acquired dyslexia (Landis, Graves, Benson, & Hebben, 1982; Moyer, 1979) have supported the use of the tactile/kinesthetic modality (letter tracing, sandpaper letters) as a temporary alternative to impaired visual pathways. While these methods may represent nothing new for special education teachers, they and other modality-specific techniques take on a new and heightened relevance for the traumatically brain damaged.

Rourke et al. (1983) suggest the use of graph paper [or ordinary lined paper turned sideways] for youngsters experiencing problems with mechanical arithmetic due to visual-spatial or graphomotor difficulties. Extra time and space, hand calculators, and tape recorders can help compensate for problems stemming from brain dysfunction. Multiple choice and matching formats for students with memory problems and oral exams for those with problems in written expression are recommended.

Simple "learning wheels" can be used to illustrate any concept that is comprised of a central focus and subordinate parts. The central focus (i.e., theme, point, goal, object) is noted in the hub of the wheel. Its secondary features (i.e., tenets, bases, steps, components) are listed on the spokes. For example, to visually embody the essence of a novel under study, the main character or premise might be noted within a circle (hub) and the answers to how, what, when, and where questions are solicited (or provided) for notation on the divergent lines (spokes). The overall product offers the THI student a coalesced and tangible representation of an otherwise vague assortment of disjointed details.

Microcomputer Programs

When carefully monitored and creatively used, microcomputer programs function as useful adjuncts to remedial programs for discrete skills that require repetition and mastery. Microcomputer programs permit students the option of working independently and promote a sense of accomplishment. They serve as an age-appropriate alternative to less stimulating worksheets and repetitive oral drill. A consistent, adjustable rate of stimulus presentation is possible, as is the automatic collection and interpretation of performance data, meaning that tedious practice tasks can be efficiently administered and objectively assessed by clinicians who are unencumbered and free to observe and supervise. Computer programs have proven to be a particularly effective means for improving attention, reaction time, visual perception and processing, reasoning and problem solving (Adamovich et al., 1985; Bolger, 1982; Gordon, Hibbard, & Kreutzer, 1989; Sohlberg & Mateer, 1989).

The major drawbacks of computer use in the rehabilitation of traumatic brain damage include their impersonal and inflexible nature and questionable utility in promoting the generalization of skills. The complications that arise as a result of THI may, in and of themselves, limit the extent to which computer use is possible. Hence, the effectiveness and suitability of software programs can not be guaranteed for all THI persons. To date, computer programs have proven least effective in the remediation of memory and language problems (Sohlberg & Mateer, 1989).

Memory Therapy

Before discussing specific techniques for improving memory, it is worth underscoring that memory performance is susceptible to and often influenced by affective states (Kahn, Zarit, Hilbert, & Niederehe, 1975). Many brain-injured individuals are sensitive to

their memory problems. This, coupled with the distress they experience as a result of being injured, can exacerbate memory problems
(Wilson & Moffat, 1984). Excessive anxiety should be reduced by
balancing deficits with a delineation of assets or by providing the
assurance that memory functions can and do improve over time.
A number of strategies can be used to make the task of remembering easier (Newcombe, 1981; Paivio, 1971; Patten, 1972; Wilson &
Moffat, 1984). One other word of caution regarding memory
dysfunction of significance to the educational as well as domestic
setting is that the act of forgetting is susceptible to reinforcement
(Wilson & Moffat, 1984). Reinforcement for forgetting often occurs
inadvertently when children or adolescents become overprotected
following an injury or are excused from responsibility. Conversely,
token reinforcement for remembering has been found to enhance
retention (Langer, Rodin, Beck, Weinman, & Spitzer, 1979). When
subjects were provided token reinforcement for remembering
predesignated information from one therapy session to the next,
their initial improvement in memory later generalized to tests of
short- and long-term memory.

Wilson and Moffat (1984) and Sohlberg and Mateer (1989) conclude that a damaged memory cannot be restored. They maintain
that the best method for helping memory-impaired individuals is
to teach the use of specific compensatory strategies that are suited
to the individual's strength and compatible with the material to be
remembered. A number of suggestions follow:

1. *Internal strategies* (mnemonics, verbal strategies, visual
   imagery)
   (a) Memory for a set of words or items (e.g., a shopping list)
       can be aided by creating an imaginary story that intercon-
       nects the words in a memorable way.
   (b) Names of people can be remembered by making a visual
       association of the person's face with an unusual feature
       and forming a verbal or visual association between the
       feature and the name.
   (c) Items can be remembered in correct order by developing
       a sentence, rhyme, acronym, or word out of the first let-
       ters of the words (e.g., the colors of the spectrum, *r*ed,
       *o*range, *y*ellow, *g*reen, *b*lue, *i*ndigo, *v*iolet can be
       remembered by the name Roy G. Biv).

(d) Rhymes or lyrics can be used to remember a set of related data such as name, age, address, date, etc. (e.g., "Albert Brown is my name. Being a brother is my game. I live on Main, at 248. For being just 10, I really rate.")

(e) For some individuals, the first letter of a word can trigger recall. Some students find that by reciting the alphabet, they can retrieve a forgotten word or name.

(f) "Chunking" is an effective means for improving serial recall (e.g., to remember a phone number, reduce the number to several chunks of two or three numerals each).

(g) "PQRST"–Glasgow et al. (1977) and Haffey (1983) demonstrated the success of this study technique with brain-injured clients. Students are guided through the strategy of previewing the order of the text or chapter; thinking of the main question to be answered by the material; reading the chapter carefully; stating the premise of what has been read; and testing for understanding.

(h) Individual items to be remembered can be "pegged" with distinct visual images such as parts of the body or rooms in a familiar house. Each visual impression is imagined and mentally linked with one of the items to be remembered.

(i) To recall an event, the visual sequence of preceding events can be recalled (i.e., the steps leading up to the forgotten event are retraced mentally).

2. *External aids* are methods used to extend or supplement internal storage mechanisms. Some examples of external aids are lists, diaries, notebooks, computers, portable timers, and electronic calculators. Various electronic signaling devices can help head-injured persons locate important personal items such as wallets, keys, or parked cars. A hard clap or whistle activates an audible homing device. Databank wristwatches are available to store names and telephone numbers. The Sharper Image Corporation carries a directory and message alarm system. Microcassette recorders can be used to record messages, reminders, notes, or instructions (Parente & Anderson-Parente, 1989). Memory-impaired clients may also be aided by means of a memory notebook (Sohlberg & Mateer, 1989). To be useful, a memory notebook should offer a practical, succinct, and efficient solution for specific memory deficits. Systematic training in the effective use of the notebook will be necessary. In concept, a memory notebook reduces memory requirements and compartmentalizes essential information. Notebook

sections are determined on the basis of individual weaknesses and situational requirements. For example, depending upon need, notebooks might include any one or more of the following sections:

(a) *orientation*—autobiographic information; details about the injury
(b) *memory log*—diary of daily events
(c) *calendar*—dates, times, appointments, schedules
(d) *things to do*—forms for recording homework assignments, errands, due dates, completion dates
(e) *transportation*—maps, bus schedules, directions
(f) *feelings log*—forms to chart feelings or reactions
(g) *names*—forms for entering names of key people
(h) *today*—necessary information to function in school, at work or home

3. *Reality Orientation Therapy (ROT).* The aim of ROT is to promote the relearning and maintenance of pertinent information such as time, place, current events, or the names of people (Wilson & Moffat, 1984). ROT incorporates such methods as verbal repetition, visual aids, behavioral training, and structured classroom conversation to improve verbal orientation. During regularly scheduled ROT sessions, individuals who have difficulty orienting themselves and remembering who, where, or how they are, are reminded of such essential information then asked to rehearse it in an informal conversation. Depending upon the student's degree of confusion or memory deficit, one or several instructional team members may schedule short reality-orientation sessions. More ideas for running effective ROT sessions can be found in Hanley (1982), Wilson and Moffat (1984), Holden and Woods (1982), and Sohlberg and Mateer (1989).

Language Therapy

Several theoretical models of language retraining seem to predominate the literature, although a sizeable number of less distinctive strategies have become equally popular (Miller, 1984). The basic tenets of the more publicized approaches to the treatment of aphasia and other noteworthy strategies will be highlighted with emphasis placed upon general principles of language therapy.

Wepman's (1951) idea of *stimulation therapy* is based on the premise that speech can be prompted by means of systematic stimulation through the use of appropriate materials and environments. Schuell, Jenkins, and Jimenez-Pabon (1964) and Taylor (1964) operationalized this approach of involving clients in a series of activities to include the simulation of everyday situations and work with classes of objects (e.g., clothing, food, animals) or groups of similar sounding words in order to stimulate speech. Extensive use of repetition and auditory stimulation by the therapist aids in prompting responses and eliciting words (Beaumont, 1983).

Operant conditioning approaches make use of the impaired individual's specific linguistic deficits. Deficit skills are task-analyzed and transformed into specific instructional objectives (Costello, 1977; Weniger, Huber, Stachowiak, & Poeck, 1980). Successive approximations are rewarded, cues are supplied then faded, and immediate feedback and reinforcement are provided (Miller, 1984).

Melodic Intonation Therapy (MIT) (Sparks, Helm, & Albert, 1974) is based upon the premise that melody is mediated by the right hemisphere. For those with relatively intact right hemispheres, singing can be used to cue deficit verbal (left-hemisphere) responses (Miller, 1984). MIT requires that short target phrases be embedded in a simple melodic pattern. The therapist encourages the client to sing phrases and sentences of increasing length in unison and then alone. This method is recommended for those with relatively intact auditory comprehension and impaired verbal expression whose expressive abilities have not responded to other forms of therapy.

Severe dysphasic individuals and those with global aphasia may require alternative communication systems (Marshall, 1989; Miller, 1984). *Visual Communication Therapy* (Gardner et al., 1976) is based upon the methods used to teach language to chimpanzees. This program, which utilizes a set of ideographic symbols for nouns, verbs, etc., has proven effective for those without oral speech. Likewise, orally apraxic individuals without speech may benefit from a format derived from the manual communication system of the North American Plains Indians, referred to as Amer-Ind (Skelly, 1979). The meanings of the signs are fairly obvious to most untrained observers. The fact that the signs can be performed with one hand makes this strategy particularly useful for hemiplegics (Miller, 1984).

Specific to the treatment of language/cognitive functions in head-injured children and adolescents, Hagen (1981) offers a set of principles for language pathologists and educational team members to follow:

1. The treatment of language disorders should be aimed at the reorganization of cognitive *processes* rather than the modification of isolated deficits.
2. Treatment stimuli should be presented through the individual's single most intact sensory modality.
3. The rate, amount, duration, and complexity of stimulus input must be manipulated in a manner that is consistent with the student's cognitive ability.
4. Treatment programs should promote the conscious processing of language in an orderly and systematic manner.

Hagen's concept of a cognitive processing hierarchy (see Table 25) offers a systematic guide for selecting and planning cognitive/language objectives. Specific treatment tasks are designed to strengthen dysfunctional and disorganized abilities. Compensatory mechanisms are taught for resistant skills (Burns, Cook, & Ylvisaker, 1988). The power of each processing skill is strengthened by increasing the rate, amount, and duration of stimulus input. The quality of each process is developed by increasing task complexity while rate, amount, and duration are held constant. Before more advanced skills are required, lower level process abilities should be well established.

When teaching traumatically brain-injured students with language-processing problems, Blosser and DePompei (1989) suggest that educators (a) pair verbal instructions with written instructions, (b) avoid figurative language, (c) provide ample time for students to process information and respond to questions, (d) illustrate critical information and key concepts with pictures and written cues, (e) vary voice and intonation when repeating instructions, and (f) define critical words and terms.

Language intervention following THI may involve environmental modifications (e.g., minimizing distractions, supplemental visual cues, increased response time); direct remediation of specific language deficits; or compensatory training. Most experts seem to agree that language therapy services should be integrated when possible (Burns et al., 1988). Integrated, as opposed to "pull out," services offer students the advantage of utilizing skills and strategies in authentic settings. Both skill generalization and maintenance are enhanced when language skills are taught and practiced in the setting where they should occur.

TABLE 25

COGNITIVE PROCESSING HIERARCHY

1. *Attention* (ability to attend to stimulus)
2. *Attention span* (ability to attend for increasing spans of time)
3. *Selective attention* (ability to suppress irrelevant stimuli)
4. *Discrimination* (ability to recognize the differences between stimuli)
5. *Temporal order, retention, and categorization* (ability to determine the whole on the basis of its parts)
6. *Association and memory* (ability to relate new information to old knowledge)
7. *Integration* (ability to integrate newly acquired knowledge with other information)
8. *Analysis and synthesis* (ability to determine the appropriate sequence of behavioral events)
9. *Execution* (ability to transmit the sequence as planned)
10. *Attention to output* (ability to attend to product)
11. *Comparison of output to intention* (ability to compare product to intention)
12. *Assessment of need for change* (ability to determine need for modifications)
13. *Modification of response* (ability to produce a modified response, if necessary)

Perceptual Retraining

Perception is involved in motor skill proficiency, sensory integration, attention, and psychological and social interactions (Abreu, 1985; Bolger, 1982). The major assumption underlying perceptual retraining is that traumatic brain injury reduces the efficiency of perceptual functions but does not necessarily result in their total eradication (Abreu, 1985). Perceptual retraining incorporates various methods aimed at improving attention, eye-hand coordination, motor planning, visual scanning, visual-spatial constructional skills, body image, awareness, and judgment (Ben-Yishay, 1980). Perceptual retraining techniques are specific to various brain systems and functions (Bolger, 1982); the recovery of perceptual functions involves the reorganization of cortical and subcortical functions (Luria, 1970a). It has been observed that individuals with right-hemisphere damage benefit from auditory stimuli and verbal strategies, whereas individuals with extensive left-hemisphere damage benefit more from visual stimuli, pantomime, demonstration, visual imagery (Diller, 1985), and melodic input (Sparks et al., 1974). This consideration of lesion laterality when selecting strategies for intervention shows the advantage of utilizing intact skills to bypass deficit skills (Diller, 1985; Luria, 1970a; Rourke et al., 1983).

At a basic level perceptual retraining promotes the stimulation and integration of auditory, visual, tactile, gustatory, olfactory, and kinesthetic functions (Adamovich et al., 1985; Ayres, 1972). It may be necessary to provide direct instruction and practice in the recognition and discrimination of color, shape, sound, and size by means of matching, sorting, ordering, categorization, and simple construction activities. Simple developmentally ordered perceptual tasks can be made more complex by increasing rate, amount, duration, and complexity of stimulus input (Hagen, 1981). In order to promote the redevelopment of perceptual skills, Hagen recommends a progressive instructional sequence for pairing input (instructional stimuli) to output (required student response); *visual* input to *visual* output (pointing, imitation, matching); *visual* to *motor* (tracing, copying, supplying the missing parts); *auditory* to *visual* (identifying the visual representation of the auditory stimulus); *auditory* to *motor* (producing a motor response to auditory stimulus); *auditory* to *verbal* (a verbal response to auditory stimulus).

Microcomputer-assisted training is a suitable complement to traditional methods of visual-perceptual rehabilitation (Lynch, 1989) such as paper-and-pencil cancellation tasks, mazes, visual closure work sheets, eye–hand coordination drills, tracing, and visual pursuit exercises. Although the advantages of computer-driven software programs as a strategic remedy for memory and language impairments are questionable, much has been written in support of computers for the remediation of deficits in visual scanning, reaction time, stimulus suppression, and tracking (Kennedy, Bittner, & Jones, 1981; Lynch, 1986; Sohlberg & Mateer, 1989).

Behavioral Management Following Traumatic Head Injury

The successful application of conventional conditioning methods with THI individuals is often limited by the neurobehavioral manifestations THI produces (Divack et al., 1985; Newcombe, 1981; Wood, 1990a). It has been well established that THI persons have difficulty reading social cues, attending, understanding cause and effect relationships, generalizing from one situation to the next, processing information, and remembering. These neural deficits can influence the degree to which conventional behavioral techniques are effective. For example, if the THI child has an impaired ability to attend to obvious environmental cues, then a behavioral strategy that presumes normal discrimination processes will undoubtedly fail. Unlike children whose brains have not been traumatized, THI children and adolescents need to experience the consequences of their behavior many times before they generalize and remember them (Barin et al., 1985). They require direct and explicit behavioral directives. Classroom rules need to be restated regularly. Behavioral treatments must be simple and persistent and delivered when and where the behavior to be modified occurs (Kazdin, 1984; Newcombe, 1981). For THI students in particular, management procedures require professional and parental collaboration, careful monitoring, and a commitment to consistency (Divack et al., 1985). The youngster should be motivated, actively involved, and aware of the program's rationale (Newcombe, 1981). In essence, behavioral management following traumatic brain injury will require (a) the manipulation of antecedent or environmental variables, or (b) a restructuring or enhancement of the consequences that follow target behaviors. To accomplish this, the practitioner will need to take into account the limitations imposed by specific neurological deficits and build in necessary adjustments.

Case Illustration

A 13-year-old female (T.N.) sustained severe craniocerebral trauma when hit by a car while biking. Following a lengthy hospital stay, she was transferred to a rehabilitation center. Within 1 month of intensive rehabilitation, her motor skills had recovered except for a mild left-sided hemiparesis. Her speech was dysarthric; she continued to experience word-finding difficulties and problems with motivation and attention. At 3 months post trauma, T.N. was still unable to sustain her attention to academic tasks for more than 5 or 6 minutes. It was decided that "time on task" would become the target behavior for modification. A bar graph was posted in the classroom and used to illustrate total time spent on task per two daily 30 minute sessions. Her parents, who visited daily, were instructed to praise her about her performance when she had either maintained or increased her time on task from the previous day. The same criterion for praise was followed by staff. By the second week of the program, she had tripled her time on task and, quite surprisingly, had improved her performance in other therapies as well. The potency of attention, social praise, and a public display of progress was well demonstrated in this case. Equally pleasing was the fact that her improved school performance had generalized to other behaviors as well. Obvious successes may have instilled the confidence she lacked and provided a momentum which generalized itself to other aspects of her program.

Intrinsic reward is often an insufficient source of reinforcement following traumatic head injury (Ince, 1976). Tangible, extrinsic rewards have been found to be far more effective (Muir et al., 1983). Without the enticement of some external motivator, many traumatically brain-injured persons will find it difficult to initiate substantial changes in their behavioral repertoires.

Case Illustration

A 16-year-old adolescent male (R.S.) was admitted for emergency treatment of severe closed head injury following a high-speed motor vehicle accident. He suffered extensive bilateral frontal lobe lesions. Nonenhanced CT scans revealed a large intraventricular hemorrhage and focal atrophy of the right frontal cortex. His initial GCS score was 4; he was comatose for approximately 3 weeks following the incident. When transferred to a rehabilitation center his behavior was marked by frequent and angry outbursts and physical aggression directed at staff. He resisted therapies, denying his need for them, and often threatened to leave the facility and "hitch a ride home." At the time, he was nonambulatory, yet fairly independent in his travel by wheelchair. Several behaviors became targets for modification, namely, his reluctance to attend therapies, lack of participation, poor attitude, and aggressiveness. The staff chose to initiate a token economy contingency management system. A gridded behavioral rating card was attached to his wheelchair. At the close of each session, his therapists rated his behavior as excellent (4 points), average (2 points), or inappropriate (0 points). The program, which was explained to R.S. at the outset, made it possible to earn between 0 and 4 points per therapy depending upon his behavior, which was judged on the basis of attendance, attitude, participation, and absence of profanity. While it was possible to earn 48 points per day, tangible reinforcement was contingent upon earning at least 35 points. Regardless of his aggregate performance, a daily meeting with a designated staff member took place for the purpose of jointly reviewing his performance, restating program goals, and (when earned) delivering a self-determined reward (he chose candy). This system, as it initially stood, was only marginally successful due to several major pitfalls: (a) Due to staff illness and schedule problems, his daily review was conducted by various staff members which interfered with the program's internal consistency; (b) Due to his limited attention span and poor memory, the client often forgot the progress (or lack thereof) he had thus far accumulated; (c) Other patients and visitors were unwittingly supplying him with candy (at his request) which seriously reduced the potency of the reinforcer. Several effective changes were made in his program: (a) *One* neutral staff member per week was assigned to carry out the day-end reviews; (b) Before and after each therapy, several minutes were taken to review the rationale of the program and the client's progress up to that time (e.g., how many points he had earned, feedback on progress, and a reminder of goals); (c) Strict enforcement of a "no candy" policy was initiated and monitored; (d) Primary rewards were delivered at a fixed interval schedule of 2 hours rather than at the end of the day. Once modified, the program produced noteworthy results. His aggressive outbursts were reduced by 50% within 2 weeks. The importance of controlling for such variables as program inconsistency, the client's cognitive liabilities, and reinforcer potency was demonstrated in this case.

Token economy systems have a fairly good history of success with brain-injured individuals (Eames, 1980; Muir et al., 1983; Sand et al., 1970; Wood, 1990a; Wood & Eames, 1981). In the school system, depending upon the individual's attention span and concentration abilities, tokens may be delivered at 15-minute or hourly intervals and later exchanged for meals (lunch), luxuries (candy, snacks, movie tickets), or privileges (early dismissal, free time).

Complex behaviors will need to be broken down into small, well-defined steps. Each step toward the target behavior should be systematically reinforced until the goal is achieved (Muir et al., 1983). Both forward and backward chaining are effective strategies for teaching a complex sequence of behaviors such as those required for eating, dressing, and other motor skills (Wood, 1990a).

Negative forms of control (time-out) have proven particularly effective for disruptive and dangerous behavior within the THI population (Muir et al., 1983; Newcombe, 1981; Sand et al., 1970;

Wood, 1987). In the school setting, an isolated room or remote corner of the classroom may provide the necessary separation from positive reinforcement (Newcombe, 1981). An important adjunct to this method, however, is the provision of positive reinforcement for cooperative and socially appropriate behavior as it occurs (Divack et al., 1985; LaVigna & Donnellan, 1986). A less drastic, yet often effective way to duplicate a temporary departure from reinforcement is to withhold social interest and attention (eye contact, involvement) or to abruptly turn away from the youngster when he/she begins to engage in mild (nondestructive, harmless) forms of inappropriate behavior (Hollon, 1973; Kazdin 1984; Newcombe, 1981).

Redirection is a particularly useful technique for interrupting perseverative behaviors. A replacement activity should be suggested to the student in a casual fashion so as not to inadvertently reinforce the inappropriate activity (Divack et al., 1985). The behavioral alternative is then immediately reinforced (Gelfand & Hartmann, 1984). Redirection is a simple but practical application of the discriminative reinforcement of other behavior (DRO). The rationale behind DRO is to increase the frequency of one (desirable) behavior in order to decrease the frequency and production of another (undesirable) behavior (Wood, 1990a).

Sometimes solutions to behavioral problems are made possible by manipulating the environment or by altering the antecedent which provokes inappropriate reactions (e.g., seating a child away from distraction, providing corrective feedback, allowing for periodic breaks from activity).

Case Illustration

A 14-year-old adolescent male (B.T.) sustained severe head injury and hypoxic brain damage when struck by a car while riding a motorcycle. Following a lengthy stay in a neurosurgical intensive care unit, he was transferred to a rehabilitation center. Upon arrival, he was grossly confused, agitated, and combative. Although capable of assisted short-distance ambulation, he was required to use a wheelchair for intertherapy travel because of his slow and unsteady gait and unpredictable behavior. His cognitive abilities were extremely impaired as a result of the injury and compounded by a global aphasia. Intermittent yet dramatic episodes of extreme agitation and combativeness began to emerge at approximately 6 months post trauma. When baseline data were established, it was evident that the target behavior (agitation/ aggression) occurred with the greatest frequency immediately following his therapies (just before he was required to return to his wheelchair). Unable to verbally communicate his distaste for wheelchair travel (and confinement in general), this young man understandably used his residual resources to make his point known. The frequency of his outbursts dramatically decreased when the wheelchair was abandoned as a means of travel. This case illustrates several critical issues: (a) the validity of environmental or antecedent control as a means of managing negative behavior; (b) the value of collecting baseline data and pinpointing the antecedents and consequences of the target behaviors; and (c) the importance of considering the client's neurological deficits and point of view.

Olson's (1983) general strategies for managing the behavior of head-injured clients provide a useful summary of the principles heretofore established. They have been modified to emphasize their applicability to the educational setting.

1. Establish the means for promoting communication among staff. Coordinate efforts to provide as consistently managed and as stable a learning environment as possible. [Regular team meetings should be scheduled to discuss student progress and, if necessary, realign or modify behavioral strategies. Between scheduled meetings, the student may be required to carry a pocket notebook so that all teachers can enter comments, behavioral ratings, or other pertinent data to be passed among staff in a reliable and timely way.]
2. Permit students to experience the logical consequences of their actions. [Repeated real-life experiences are much more potent than verbal reprimands which are often too abstract to be understood and remembered.]
3. Separate long-term goals into small sequential steps to promote success and reduce frustration.
4. Provide clear and direct feedback regarding behaviors. [Direct statements such as "Jim, please sit in your chair" are more effective than subtle and nondescript innuendos.]
5. Model calm, controlled, and predictable behavior.
6. Provide environmental compensations to reduce stress and counter negative behaviors. [Provide periodic breaks during the day, pace demands, minimize distractions, and maintain

a flexible structure. Two 15-minute sessions are often much more productive than one continuous 30-minute span.]

7. Redirect rather than confront perseverative and organically based behaviors, such as redundancy, response sets, and compulsive tendencies. [Involve student in a replacement activity that is incompatible with the undesired behavior.]

8. Expect variable performance from THI students. Modify expectations accordingly.

9. Set reasonable expectations that take into account the age of the individual, the extent of dysfunction, and potential for recovery.

10. Involve the family in the behavioral management plan.

Specialized Psychological and Psychiatric Interventions

Individual Counseling

The predominant psychological issue faced by those who have experienced traumatic injury is loss (Castelnuovo-Tedesco, 1984). For THI individuals who are cognitively aware, the feelings of personal loss are common (Barin et al., 1985). They may mourn the loss of body, mind, function, mobility, or specific hopes for the future (Krueger, 1984; Lezak, 1978). Reactions to traumatic head injury are likely to follow the same course as do reactions to other significant losses of a personal nature (e.g., the loss of someone loved). Initial shock, denial, and depression typically precede acceptance and adaptation (Kubler-Ross, 1969). In an attempt to avoid the anxiety, depression, and psychic pain associated with their accident and injury, THI persons may develop any number of defensive reactions such as avoidance, passivity, denial, displacement, uncontrollable behavior, or projection (Krueger, 1984). Coping, on the other hand, involves the process of reasonable and advantageous adaptation (Krueger, 1984). It is toward this goal of reasonable and advantageous adaptation that counseling with THI children and adolescents should be focused. Helping head-injured persons accept their trauma, its consequences, and their new circumstances is a challenge to all responsible for their educational programming. Individual and/or group counseling services can offer a source of acceptance and support, realistic feedback, and a safe atmosphere for practicing and relearning appropriate interpersonal skills (Barin et al., 1985). Some students may need an explanation of traumatic head injury or assistance in developing ways to compensate for their acquired inadequacies. The developmental stage of an individual at the point of traumatic injury will influence his/her perception of it (Tarnow, 1984). For example, adolescents are more apt to show such responses as suicidal depression, loss of self-esteem, denial, and irresponsible behavior, whereas younger children are likely to develop associated fears, separation anxiety, guilt, and acting-out behaviors (Barin et al., 1985; Blazyk, 1983).

Tarnow (1984) provides some direction for practitioners in a position to counsel with children and adolescents struggling with acquired handicaps:

1. Deal with the initial circumstances, i.e., the injury, the disability.
2. [Promote] as normal a pattern of development as possible.
3. Prevent maladaptive (defensive) mechanisms from taking root.
4. Plan and institute short-term, middle-range, and long-term rehabilitative [goals] specific to the individual's and family's needs.
5. Develop a therapeutic plan to modify body image and problems with self-esteem.
6. Help the individual maintain contact and an active exchange with the environment and social context.
7. Promote the individual's development of special skills according to abilities.
8. Help the individual work through fantasies of what caused the condition and bring into consciousness the fact that it was not punishment for misdeeds or bad thoughts.
9. Build on strengths incorporating vocational counseling early in adolescence.
10. Provide parent counseling to prevent passive dependence and overprotection. Parent groups are suggested.
11. For adolescents, issues of sexuality, identity, autonomy, and peer group relations may be dealt with in a group format.
12. Counsel with staff members and peers in order to counteract their tendency to provoke maladaptive mechanisms.
13. Conduct periodic evaluations so that signs of fixation or psychological regression can be detected. Psychotherapy is advised when these symptoms persist.

Psychotherapy

Until recently, psychotherapy has not been considered a viable intervention for the traumatically brain-injured. Impaired cognitive,
communication, and memory functions have been viewed as major
obstacles to meaningful gain via psychotherapy. Lewis (1991) views
the reluctance of therapists to treat brain-injured clients as having
more to do with the therapist than the client. She contends that
many therapists tend to overestimate the differences between brain-
injured and neurologically intact individuals and underestimate the
similarities both populations share. If the broad goals of psychotherapy are to help clients clarify misconceptions, correct faulty
beliefs about the self, increase awareness of repressed feelings, and
gain self-control (Prigatano, 1991), then brain-injured individuals
should be considered no less suited and no less entitled to its potential benefits than the neurologically intact. The pathology for which
psychotherapy is ordinarily recommended to neurologically intact
individuals (e.g., disordered cognition, faulty self-perceptions,
maladaptive behaviors, denial, and limited self-control) has, by
contrast, an "organic" basis following traumatic brain injury.
Although this distinction of organicity need not alter the broad aims
of psychotherapy, it does call for modification in the process by and
context within which therapy is provided. Prigatano (1991)
eloquently describes these essential adjustments from practical,
individual, and neuropsychological perspectives. In a practical sense,
therapists can best assist by developing an understanding of the
client's experiences and resistances and helping him or her actively
engage in the rehabilitation process. Cicerone (1991) recommends
unconditional validation of the client's perceptions initially, followed
by the gradual reconciliation of discrepancies between perceptions,
reality, and expectations. The client's personal symbols of work, love,
and play may be used as the basis for reassigning meaning to life
(Prigatano, 1991). With guidance, unrealistic symbols are examined
and the obstacles to productivity and satisfying interpersonal relationships are tactfully confronted. Successful execution of the
aforementioned strategies will depend upon the accommodations
made for neuropsychological residua (Lewis, 1991). Problems with
abstract reasoning and communication will require the use of novel
and creative strategies. Music, art, literature, and storytelling can

help clients with brain injury formulate their inner experiences through external means (Prigatano, 1991) and ease the burden placed upon deficit functions. Memory problems may be accommodated by increasing the frequency of sessions and limiting topics to one or two per session. Frequent repetition of key concepts and the requirement of oral or written summaries after each session can enhance learning and retention (Lewis, 1991).

In addition to the procedural modifications required to address neurologic and cognitive deficits, Lewis (1991) identifies three issues that merit equal attention and proper assessment if one is to optimize the impact of psychotherapy following traumatic brain injury, namely, (a) the psychological meaning and impact of the deficit upon the patient, (b) the psychological factors that exist independent of the injury, and (c) the broader social context. When the therapist understands the meaning and impact of the deficits from the client's point of view, he or she is better equipped to distinguish among various motives and can plan treatment accordingly. For example, answers to the following questions will help direct the course and emphasis of therapy. Are the symptoms exaggerated for the purpose of secondary gain such as a release from responsibility? Are they tied to premorbid feelings of victimization? Do they serve a protective function or are they purely reactive in nature (Christensen & Rosenberg, 1991)?

When formulating treatment plans, the client's premorbid character and ego functioning should also be assessed. Issues that were unresolved prior to the injury, although likely to continue in exaggerated form after the injury, are of an independent nature. Such analysis helps elucidate the distinction between organically based and characterological disorders. Furthermore, the careful assessment of preinjury behavioral patterns and intact personality structures provides a basis for predictions and the means by which to develop realistic interventions.

The broader social context that entails family, roles, structures, and alliances; level of emotional support; economic stability; and expectations will have a strong influence upon treatment approaches and the impact of psychotherapy. Given the dynamics of the survivor's social network, it may be useful to involve others in the therapeutic process.

Videotherapy and Interpersonal Process Recall (IPR)

The advantages of video as a therapeutic tool for use with the THI population are rather striking when one considers the types of cognitive, behavioral, and social problems that commonly beset these individuals, such as, poor interpersonal skills, memory deficit, problems in reading social cues, diminished self-concept, and communication problems. The value of providing clients with an immediate visual and audio representation of their behavior has been highly promoted (Kagan, 1975) and clearly described by Heilveil (1983) in her book *Video in Mental Health Practice*. A wealth of novel themes and specific strategies are included in her text along with general guidelines for individual and group treatments. Heilveil highlights the value of video in various treatment milieus (i.e., individual counseling and therapy with children and adolescents, group and family work, within the classroom) and its usefulness in the treatment of hyperactivity, low self-esteem, depression, and social incompetence. It can be used to help clients (a) prepare for job interviews, (b) develop effective interpersonal strategies, (c) model effective behaviors, (d) reduce annoying behaviors and mannerisms, or (e) practice a feared social encounter. Before using video equipment in therapy with children and adolescents, it is necessary to obtain written permission and advisable to discuss the purposes of videotaping. The tapes should be erased when they no longer serve a therapeutic purpose and the client should be informed of this (Heilveil, 1983).

Interpersonal Process Recall (IPR) is a specific videotaping strategy which was originated by Norman Kagan in the early 1960's. (The film package "Influencing Human Interaction" which details the use of IPR is available from Mason Media, Inc., Box C, Mason, MI 48854.) The IPR technique was originally developed as a means for improving skills of human interaction and communication. Kagan (1969, 1975) noted that if an individual was videotaped while relating to another person and immediately shown the recording, his/her ability to recall thoughts and feelings was greatly enhanced. Kagan and Krathwohl (1967) found that this process could be further enhanced if the client had the assistance of someone who would encourage elaboration and recall during the viewing phase. The best results were achieved when the "facilitator" focused on underlying thoughts and feelings as opposed to confrontation and critique. Helffenstein (1981) found evidence that IPR was an effective means for improving the interpersonal skills of traumatically brain-injured adolescents and young adults. As part of his study, he identified a number of useful follow-up questions that were effective in stimulating thought, communicativeness, and insight:

- How did that make you feel?
- What were you thinking at the time?
- What were you imagining at that point?
- What did you want to hear?
- What do you think he/she was thinking about you?
- What else did you want to say?
- What do you think he/she was trying to tell you?
- What would you do differently? How would you change?

Follow-up questions are used to (a) inspire affective exploration and cognitive examination; (b) formulate expectations, perceptions, desired images; (c) develop skill in reading nonverbal cues; and (d) permit the learning and practice of new methods and styles of interaction. Because interpersonal effectiveness, communication, and the ability to benefit from traditional forms of social feedback are frequently compromised by THI, the unique combination of technology (videotaping) and human guidance (facilitator) of IPR makes it a powerful treatment tool with many possible applications (Helffenstein, 1981). Because of its inherent flexibility, IPR can be used to improve social eye contact and memory skills, develop conversational skills, enhance self-concept, improve posture, and reduce social anxieties. THI individuals with severe aphasia, visual or hearing problems are not appropriate candidates for IPR.

The basic format of IPR requires that the client be videotaped while engaged in an interaction with another professional (e.g., counselor, speech pathologist, teacher). The individual with whom the client interacted may or may not be involved in the review (mutual recall), during which time the facilitator assists the client in evaluating and understanding personal thoughts, feelings, and behaviors. The facilitator (e.g., school psychologist, guidance counselor, speech pathologist, special education teacher) keeps a brief log of deficits observed and skills facilitated. Although acceptable results can be achieved with less, in its purest form, the IPR process calls for at least two rooms, two video cameras, and a special-effects generator capable of creating a split-screen image (Heilveil, 1983). One room serves as a studio for videotaping and recall sessions; the second room is equipped for viewing and recording recall sessions. In the studio, each camera is focused upon one of the participants from opposite corners of the room. The special-effects generator blends the two images for later viewing. A modified version of the IPR process using one strategically placed camera and one room has produced acceptable results (V. Westervelt, personal communication, 1986), although the technological product is less refined.

Case Illustration

A 10-year-old male (L.T.) sustained a severe closed head injury (GCS = 4) when involved in a motor vehicle accident. Early CT scans (nonenhanced) revealed a left intracranial hemorrhage in the thalamic region. An EEG revealed left-sided multifocal evidence of seizure activity. Some decerebrate posturing was noted along with elevated ICP. At 1 month post injury, L.T. was transferred to a pediatric rehabilitation center still comatose (GCS = 8). Within 3 months of the trauma, L.T. was ambulatory, but exhibited an unusual gait and poor balance. Short-term memory deficits, slow visual-motor processing speed, poor fine motor control, low volume monotone speech, poor concentration skills, mild ataxia, poor eye contact, and moderate depression were also present. An *eclectic* format that combined the technological advantages of videotaping, the theoretical aspects of role playing, and the salient features of IPR were used to facilitate improvement in this youngster's interpersonal skills (Westervelt & Rozzi, 1985). The behaviors targeted for potential modification were his poor short-term memory, poor eye contact, low-volume and monotone speech, and poor social confidence. Four similar 40-minute sessions were conducted over a 3-week span according to the following format:

1. *Initial interview.* Client and interviewer were videotaped while engaged in a 5–10-minute therapeutic interview. The facilitator (therapist) remained in the room but out of the client's view.
2. *Focus replay.* The facilitator joined the client and the interviewer adjourned. Facilitator and client reviewed the tape which was stopped by the facilitator (or client) for comment and inspection.

3. *Assessment*. The client's reactions to the presentation were discussed. Problem areas were first identified by the client (in this case, poor posture, fleeting eye contact, low-volume speech). The facilitator restated the client's appraisal and suggested role play.
4. *Behavioral rehearsal*. With the targeted behaviors in mind, the client and facilitator were taped engaging in a 5–10-minute role play session, wherein the client rehearsed and modified his behavior according to plan.
5. *Performance feedback and recall*. Both facilitator and interviewer assisted client in identifying behavioral improvements and modifications. Positive feedback was provided for client's attempts to modify behavior. Gentle but assertive prodding was used to help client disclose underlying motivations, expectations and feelings about his transformed behaviors.

For a number of reasons, this combined strategy became an efficient and effective catalyst for improving this youngster's interpersonal skills. L.T. was particularly motivated to regain his former image and was capable of facing evidence of his losses. Secondly, the child and his facilitator had been able to develop a sound and therapeutic relationship prior to the initiation of videotherapy. While formal measures of pre- and posttreatment behavior were not taken, subjective evidence of its effectiveness was based upon (a) immediate visual evidence of increased eye contact, improved posture, and vocal inflection during the first session; (b) subsequent unsolicited remarks by staff and relatives that his interpersonal and communicative skills had improved; (c) testimony by the child that change had occurred to his satisfaction; and (d) a videotaped follow-up at 6 months which illustrated that interpersonal changes had been maintained.

Social Skills Training

To meet the challenge of reestablishing social competency in THI children and adolescents, direct and structured skills training is recommended. The efficacy of social skills training following THI has been confirmed (Hopewell et al., 1990). The step-by-step approach promoted in most social skills training programs when augmented by demonstration, role play, practice exercises, repetitiveness, and generalization training is exactly "what the doctor should order" for children with executive dysfunction, memory problems, aggressiveness, and social ineptness. Gresham (1981) identifies three common reasons why children fail to engage in pro-social behaviors: (a) *skill deficits* (the child may not know what the appropriate behavior is); (b) *performance deficits* (the child may have the skill, but may lack practice); and (c) *self-control deficits* (emotional responses may inhibit skill performance). Organically based variations of the above themes seem to be equally applicable to the traumatically brain-injured. Damaged cognitive and personality functions can result in an impaired ability to interpret social cues, disorganized cognitive processes, disinhibition, poor initiation skills, poor self-correction ability, poor judgment, or poor interpersonal skills.

The structured learning approach (Goldstein et al., 1980) is a useful format for teaching social skills to THI children and adolescents. The four components of the structured learning approach follow.

1. The target skill is first demonstrated by the trainer. (MODEL-ING)
2. Trainees are given the opportunity to practice the skill. (ROLE PLAY)
3. Trainees are provided immediate feedback on the adequacy of their performance. (PERFORMANCE FEEDBACK)
4. Trainees are encouraged to practice and use the skill in real life. (TRANSFER OF TRAINING)

Social skills training efforts may be individualized for THI students by means of cue cards, reinforcement schedules, videotaping, relaxation training, visual cues attached to notebooks for in vivo reference, increased emphasis upon generalization and maintenance activities, and follow-up booster sessions (Hopewell et al., 1990).

Psychiatric Intervention

As a rule, psychiatric interventions for the THI child and adolescent are more likely to be rendered during the acute stages of recovery than during middle and late stages. In some instances, however, late-onset emotional disorders do develop, for which psychiatric intervention and medication may be required. Barin et al. (1985) identify five late-onset conditions for which psychiatric consultation may be necessary.

1. *To treat extreme agitation and emotional lability.* Tricyclic antidepressants have been successful in stabilizing emotional lability, although they have a tendency to lower the convulsive thresholds in those not receiving anticonvulsant therapy (Mysiw & Jackson, 1987; Peck, Stern, & Watkinson, 1983). The full therapeutic effect of antidepressants, however, may not be evident until maximal doses have been taken for a period of 6 weeks (Glenn & Wroblewski, 1989). Barin et al. (1985) contend that in extreme cases of severe agitation and emotional lability, the advantages of drug treatment far outweigh the dangers. Antipsychotic medications (e.g., Mellaril, Haldol, Thorazine) have been used to treat self-injurious bouts of agitation, extreme hostility, and physical aggression yet have been found to inhibit the return of cognitive function (Cardenas, 1987; Cope, 1986; Feeney, Gonzalez, & Law, 1982).

2. *To intervene in severe depressive reactions.* The incidence of depression following traumatic brain injury may be as high as 65% (Cicerone, 1991). Suicidal threats and self-injurious behavior will require immediate and sustained treatment. For some children and adolescents, medication may be necessary.

3. *To motivate severely impaired persons to use their residual abilities.* A loss of hope and the onset of depression generally accompany motivational problems. Other THI survivors can be particularly effective in motivating discouraged individuals by personal example. Overly sympathetic attitudes, however, tend to undermine the confidence and optimism of THI persons. Barin et al. (1985) advocate a gentle yet firm approach on the part of the treatment staff. When staff efforts fail to promote appreciable gain, psychiatric or psychopharmacological intervention should be explored.

4. *To treat psychotic reactions.* Although psychotic reactions are rare following head injury, a mild disorganized psychosis may develop (Cardenas, 1987). Small doses of antipsychotic medications (also called neuroleptics) that do not cause sedation (e.g., Trilafon, Prolixin, or Stelazine) have been recommended when psychotherapy fails. One drawback of such medication, however, is its negative impact upon cognitive function (Cope, 1986, 1987).

5. *To address the reemergence of premorbid personality disorders or psychiatric problems.* As the recovery process unfolds, preexisting psychiatric problems, substance abuse, or related character disorders may resurface. Intensive counseling, strict enforcement of rules

regarding illegal possession, referral to Alcoholics or Narcotics Anonymous, and other conventional methods may be useful, providing the individual is psychologically capable of cooperating. Failure to respond to these interventions may warrant psychiatric consultation or referral.

Psychopharmacological Intervention

A modern text on traumatic brain injury would not be complete without some mention of recent trends in psychopharmacology. The coverage to follow is by no means exhaustive or absolute. For up-to-date information when evaluating drug applications for specific clinical circumstances, additional sources will need to be consulted. Those interested in further preliminary reading are directed to the articles of Cardenas, 1987, Cope, 1987, Evans and Gualtieri, 1987, Glenn and Joseph, 1987, Glenn and Wroblewski, 1989, Gualtieri, 1991, Horn, 1987, Joshi, Capozzoli, and Coyle, 1985, Parmelee and O'Shanick, 1987.

The suitability of pharmacological approaches in the treatment of psychiatric conditions, not unlike that of most treatment methods initiated following THI, depends upon the patient's specific physiologic state and characteristics, premorbid variables, and personality structure. For the most part, much of what is known about the applicability of pharmacological methods for the THI population has been derived from animal research or empirical and scientific studies of other, often unrepresentative, patient groups. Hence, sufficient data have not yet accumulated to support broad and transferrable drug applications for the traumatically brain injured (Cope, 1987). The extent to which pathology and the physiologic states of brain-injured persons resemble those whose neurologic makeup has not been altered is unclear.

Without the advantage of scientific corroboration, the potential for misuse and unanticipated complications exists. Misuse occurs when medication is insufficiently monitored, used to compensate for inadequate staff, or relied upon as a convenient alternative to less invasive and potentially successful strategies. THI individuals are by nature often limited in their ability to give informed consent (Haas, 1987). Furthermore, the long-term cost of rehabilitation following THI has prompted a rationing of treatment applications, which has led to an almost exclusive reliance upon traditional, though not necessarily optimal, methodologies. In sum, the pharmacological treatment of behavioral and psychiatric complications following THI is beset with ethical, legal, and economic constraints.

Although pharmacological intervention cannot undo the primary damage that results from THI, it has the potential to alter the cerebral environment physiologically and to remedy deficit neurological activity in ways not possible by standard rehabilitation approaches (Cope, 1987; Evans & Gualtieri, 1987). No pharmaceutical agent, however, works with maximal efficiency, effectiveness, and minimal side effects in all persons. The multiple events that take place following THI (axonal tearing, hypoxic complications, damage due to increased intracranial pressure, focal lesions) unpredictably influence the effects of neuroactive agents (Cope, 1987). Unless the potential advantages of pharmacological intervention outweigh the disadvantages (viz., a counterproductive influence upon recovery, exacerbation of other more serious complications, sensory-motor or cognitive dulling), drug use has typically been avoided in favor of other less invasive strategies such as behavior management, cognitive rehabilitation, psychotherapy, and so forth (Chamovitz et al., 1985; Feeney et al., 1982; Sutton, Weaver, & Feeney, 1987). Emerging research indicates, however, that antipsychotics, antidepressants, stimulants, beta blockers, and an assortment of atypical medications are being used with increasing frequency in the successful treatment of such posttraumatic symptoms as paranoia, mental confusion, severe agitation, aggression, depression, attention deficits, hypertension, seizure disorders, and memory problems (Cardenas, 1987; Cassidy, 1990; Cope, 1990; Evans & Gualtieri, 1987; Horn, 1987; Mysiw & Jackson, 1987; O'Shanick, 1987).

Stimulant Medication. The therapeutic effectiveness of psychostimulant compounds for disorders of attention is remarkably well established. As a result, psychostimulants are being used with increasing frequency to treat the attentional problems associated with traumatic brain injury. Evans and Gualtieri (1987) consider the behavioral, psychologic, and cognitive symptoms of THI and attention deficit hyperactivity disorder (ADHD) to be similar on clinical grounds. Thus, the comparable efficacy of stimulant medication in the treatment of THI children and adolescents is not surprising. Stimulants in low to moderate doses have been found to counter the problems of distractibility, hyperactivity, impulsiveness, and excitability, as well as poor attention, emotional lability, slow perceptual motor speed, and memory. Anecdotal data seem to support the long-term clinical efficacy and safety of stimulant treatment following THI (Weinstein & Wells, 1981).

The possible short-term effects of stimulant medication include anorexia and insomnia. These effects often subside in time or with dose adjustments. Headaches and stomach aches are more common and may warrant discontinuation of the drug. Irritability and dysphoria or depression often coincide with the initiation of treatment or, alternately, appear after prolonged use (Evans & Gualtieri, 1987). Stimulants raise, not lower, seizure thresholds. Perseveration and stereotypic behavior are usually high-dose responses. Dyskinesias (uncontrollable body movement and tics) have been reported to occur following stimulant treatment. THI children and adolescents with severe motor impairments are less likely to respond favorably and appear to be more sensitive to toxic effects and withdrawal reactions (Evans & Gualtieri, 1987).

Family Counseling

The unexpected social and psychological complications brought about by a traumatic head injury can produce profound and lasting effects upon family functioning. A family's sense of equilibrium, its rules, routines, power structures, alliances, financial stability, and communication patterns can undergo considerable change when one member sustains a life-altering head injury (DePompei & Zarski, 1989). A family's ability to adjust to the effects of head trauma is highly dependent upon (a) the perceptions each member maintains about changes in the patient, (b) the patient's developmental stage, (c) the patterns of family interaction prior to the injury, and (d) the strategies and resources the family uses to cope and reorganize (Minuchin, 1974; Zarski, DePompei, West, & Hall, 1988). The adjustment reactions and stages through which family systems proceed vary, although generally follow the pattern of (a) shock, (b) denial, (c) anxiety, (d) anger, (e) realization, (f) retreat, (g) depression, (h) acknowledgment, and (i) acceptance (Kubler-Ross, 1969; Rollin, 1984). In their quest for resolution, it is not uncommon for family members to resort to any one or more of the following coping strategies (DePompei & Zarski, 1989):

Suppression — the tendency to remain distant from central issues (e.g., greater concern about what the child will wear to school rather than about the child's school program, issues of staff preparation, or the child's ability to progress).

Avoidance/Denial — refusing to acknowledge the presence of problems, expressing the belief that all will return to normal once the child returns home. Avoidance and denial reactions may also take the form of rescuing, i.e., protecting the child from the natural consequences of his or her actions.

Projection — projecting unacceptable impulses or feelings onto the child or other family members.

Regression — reverting to behaviors that may have been useful at an earlier stage (e.g., treating or talking to the injured child as though he or she were much younger).

Displacement — displacing angry feelings about the injured child on someone else (e.g., the parent may feel angry at the child for becoming injured but because anger is perceived as an unacceptable feeling under the circumstances, it is displaced on someone else).

Some families adjust to the stresses associated with traumatic brain injury by reacting with normal expressions of grief. They eventually acknowledge the limitations of the disabled member and come to accept the limits of their own resources. As a result, these "functional" families are able to resume involvement in other aspects of their lives (Klonoff & Prigatano, 1987).

Dysfunctional families, by contrast, become consumed by the disability and its unfairness. An inordinate amount of time is spent either blaming themselves or the head injury survivor. Family members may experience extreme difficulty accepting and accommodating alterations in the character and personality brought about by the brain injury. Impairments are denied, professional help is often rejected, and unrealistic goals for recovery are rigidly maintained. Rosenthal and Muir (1983) identify three patterns of family functioning that place families at serious risk for counterproductive reactions: (a) a premorbid history of family problems such as marital discord or alcoholism; (b) an extensive period of denial; and (c) severe and prolonged cognitive or physical impairment in the injured child. Families who exhibit these at-risk characteristics and those showing obvious signs of enmeshment (overinvolvement), disengagement (lack of concern), or extreme rigidity should be offered therapeutic counseling.

Family counseling following head injury is best accomplished by a clinician who is both comfortable and familiar with the dynamics of traumatic brain injury (Cicerone, 1991; Lezak, 1978). The focus of treatment should be aimed at enabling family members to experience the necessary reactions to their grief. Members of the family should be encouraged to develop useful response patterns whenever feasible. Productive responses may need to be modeled. When providing critical information to the head injury survivor and family, it is wise to request that the information conveyed be restated at strategic intervals to check for accuracy and understanding. Predictions about recovery should be offered with sensitivity and candor.

Counseling efforts should (a) help family members set realistic expectations, (b) provide guidance in behavioral management and parent effectiveness, and (c) direct family members toward an awareness of their needs and their responsibilities to themselves and to one another (Blazyk, 1983; Overs & Healy, 1973; Polinko, 1985). Family members need not feel guilty when their care does not result in improvements (Lezak, 1978). They may also need to hear that frustration, anger, and sorrow are natural responses to the serious injury of a loved one. Parents should be encouraged to take care of themselves first if they are to continue giving optimum care to their son or daughter (Lezak, 1978).

Within the educational setting, a well-informed school psychologist can assist the family by (a) securing, relaying, and interpreting significant cognitive, psychological, neuropsychological, and behavioral information to school personnel prior to the child's reentry; (b) assisting in the development of an appropriate treatment plan; (c) providing ongoing consultation to staff and information on the nature and consequences of traumatic head injury; (d) regularly monitoring student progress to document changes; (e) interpreting such changes as indicative of real improvement, appropriate versus inappropriate program or treatment strategies, regression, or psychological variables; (f) providing individual or group counseling to promote advantageous adjustment; and (g) providing family counseling, behavioral consultation, and/or referral.

11

EDUCATIONAL PROGRAM PLANNING AND REINTEGRATION FOLLOWING TRAUMATIC HEAD INJURY

To realistically plan and implement meaningful educational treatment programs for head-injured students, an understanding of the complexities of THI is essential (Savage & Carter, 1984). The unique characteristics of THI individuals make it necessary for professionals to actively prepare for their return to school. Given the many demands placed upon practitioners who interface with the special education process and who deal with the issues of nontraditional programming, it is indeed difficult to find time to go beyond the limits of what is routinely mandated. With respect to the traumatically brain injured, however, the time taken to prepare for their return to public school and to learn about the nature of head trauma, the recovery course, associated sequelae, and the specific changes a student has undergone will be time well spent. The alternative to a state of preparedness may well be the expenditure of considerably more time in trying to impose structure on a hopelessly disorganized and frustrating situation. With an understanding of THI, the directions to take and strategies to impose are more clearly and easily recognized. In essence, those responsible for reintegration are in a position to speak the same language and able to promote appropriate program components on a more informed, efficient, and unified basis.

Head injuries can produce any combination of physical, mental, and social by-products. For this reason, treatment becomes the responsibility of many specialists. The interdisciplinary approach characteristic of the rehabilitative model can be duplicated within the public school system when school psychologist, speech pathologist, learning specialists, social worker/counselor, adaptive physical education teacher, occupational/physical therapist, school nurse, regular classroom teacher, vocational counselor, and parents join forces to develop a suitable program. Moreover, many of the strategies used in rehabilitation centers can be adapted for use within the educational setting.

A student's readiness to re-enter the public schools is largely determined on the basis of medical discharge criteria such as physical and medical stability or behavioral manageability. Medical readiness for discharge does not guarantee readiness for the demands of the public school. Cohen and coworkers (1985) consider the following prerequisites necessary if one is to benefit from a school experience: an ability to

1. attend to task for 10 to 15 minutes;
2. tolerate 20 to 30 minutes of typical classroom stimulation (noises, movement, distractions, etc.);
3. function within a group of two or more students;
4. follow simple directions (written, verbal, or gestural);
5. engage in some type of meaningful communication (talking, pointing, communication device, or gaze); and
6. evidence some degree of learning potential.

Preparing for Student Re-entry

During the initial stages of a child's hospitalization, medical staff will need to rely upon school personnel for educational histories, preinjury assessment data for purposes of comparison, school books, and class assignments. Prior to discharge, rehabilitation personnel may need to visit the THI child's home and school to assess physical layout, architectural barriers, and potential hazards. During the interim, progress reports and ongoing communication with public school staff should be maintained (Ylvisaker, Hartwick, & Stevens, 1991). Preliminary meetings between school and rehabilitation staff greatly ease and enhance the reintegration process. The importance of coordinating reintegration efforts with the referring hospital or rehabilitation center is not to be underestimated. Medical staff can provide school personnel with specific recommendations, consultation, and comprehensive multidisciplinary discharge summaries. Medical, educational, sociological, physical, occupational, speech/language, and recreational therapy summaries, along with psychological and neuropsychological evaluations, should be collected and reviewed in preparation for the student's return. Table 26 includes 20 objectives for medical treatment teams to pursue in preparation for the transition process. Table 27 contains 20 questions school personnel should have answered prior to the THI student's return. These questions can be used to organize the data-gathering process or may serve as a format for interviewing medical personnel; the answers will help predict service, instructional, and programming needs.

In most cases, the THI student's eligibility for special education services will need to be determined and, if eligible, an individualized education program (IEP) developed (see Table 28 for sample preliminary service plan/IEP for THI students). Related services such as special transportation, counseling, or specialized therapies may be necessary. IEP goals for THI students should focus on the remediation of deficit skills that interfere with educational progress and independent functioning, functions amenable to improvement, and areas that if remediated or circumvented (by means of compensatory training) would open up new avenues for learning.

Because rapid recovery can take place during the early postinjury stages, 2 or 3 weeks of added recovery time can warrant major changes in educational plans. Some school systems have found it useful to delay final placement decisions until the student can be observed in the classroom setting. During the early stages of reentry, many THI students will require close supervision and monitoring of their whereabouts, particularly at the secondary level. They may need direction during firedrills and structure during periods of free time and low supervision (Boll, 1983). Some may be better assigned to the guidance department or resource room rather than study hall. At the secondary level, the guidance counselor is usually in the best position to coordinate the academic program and communicate with teachers on a daily basis so that disorganization and potential manipulation by the student is kept in check. Counselors or resource teachers may serve as a student's primary contact person with whom he/she "checks in" and "out" each day.

Decisions about drivers' education need to be made with the adolescent's physician or neuropsychologist and parents on the basis

TABLE 26

PLANNING FOR RE-ENTRY:
TWENTY OBJECTIVES FOR MEDICAL TREATMENT TEAMS

Initially
1. Establish key school and medical contacts.
2. Collect formal and informal records of child's preinjury status. Request school books and assignments.
3. Establish parameters of child's former school day, routines, and curriculum.
4. Begin informal discussion of THI and possible outcomes.
5. Discuss program/placement options and range of ancillary services available.

During Admission
6. Provide regular update on progress and projected program and service needs.
7. Arrange for school and hospital on-site visits for medical and educational treatment teams.
8. Assess school's physical layout and potential barriers.
9. Determine need for inservice training, consultation, and/or peer preparation.
10. Discuss projected re-entry time frame.
11. Prepare family for the school re-entry process and child's projected service needs.
12. Conduct multidisciplinary assessment at Rancho Level VI or during last month of hospitalization (see Table 18 "Format for Organizing and Reporting")
13. Refer for special education services, if appropriate.
14. Establish requirements for and date of school's eligibility meeting.
15. Forward medical, psychological, educational, sociocultural, and specialized therapy evaluation summaries at least 2 to 3 weeks prior to anticipated discharge. Provide videotape of recommended behavioral management, therapeutic, and instructional techniques.

Prior to Discharge
16. Participate in school's eligibility meeting and IEP development.
17. Facilitate identified inservice training, consultation, and peer preparation needs.
18. Determine child's school-based re-entry case manager.
19. Participate in the coordination of school and community-based services and/or outpatient therapy.
20. Establish follow-up schedule and postdischarge contacts.

of seizure status, visual acuity and perception, judgment, and motor control (Rosen & Gerring, 1986). Jones, Giddens, and Croft (1983) recommend that the training of brain-damaged drivers involve the expertise of an occupational therapist who can assist staff in measuring visual status, reaction timing, tracking, and assessing relative medical and psychological fitness. The Cognitive Behavioral Driver's Inventory has been developed to assist with the standardized

TABLE 27

PLANNING FOR RE-ENTRY:
TWENTY QUESTIONS FOR EDUCATIONAL TREATMENT TEAMS

1. What type of injury did the child sustain? (open or closed)
2. What was the extent of damage? (mild, moderate, severe)
3. What areas of the brain were compromised?
4. How long was the child unconscious?
5. When did the injury occur? How old was the child at the time?
6. What was the child's estimated cognitive and educational status before the injury?
7. How long after the injury was assessment conducted?
8. What notable sensory impairments does the child exhibit?
9. What motor impairments prevail and how will this impact the child's ability to function within the academic setting?
10. What are the child's predominant cognitive, physical, academic, and/or behavioral problems?
11. What are the child's strengths? Which functions remain intact?
12. How long is the child's attention span?
13. What specialized equipment will the child need?
14. What personal assistance will the child require?
15. Does the child require medication?
16. Is the child at risk for seizures?
17. What safety precautions need to be taken?
18. What special concerns do the child's parents have?
19. Can the child's needs be addressed within the regular classroom?
20. Does the child qualify for special education and ancillary services?

assessment of operational driving skills in brain-injured clients (Engum & Lambert, 1990). Informed decisions should also be made about career and vocational plans (Bolton, 1982; Tufts Medical Center, 1984). Former goals may need to be reassessed and action taken to redirect academic and vocational pursuits. A complete and timely vocational assessment is recommended when new direction is needed (Musante, 1983; Silver & Kay, 1989; Smith, 1983).

The transition from hospital to home and school is a stressful adjustment for most children and adolescents. The return to school spotlights personal losses, specifically the cognitive, physical, academic, and social changes that have taken place. IDEA entitles THI youngsters to an appropriate education and requires that

TABLE 28
PRELIMINARY SERVICE PLAN/IEP FOR THI STUDENTS

Student Name _____ School _____
Initial IEP Date _____ IEP Review _____

Summary of Present
Level of Performance

Projected Long-term Goals

Projected Short-term Objectives	Specific Strategies and/or Support Services	Persons Responsible	Begin/ Review

Percent Time in Regular Classroom	Trial Placement Recommendation

Committee Recommendations for Specific Procedures/Techniques (include information about learning style, compensatory devices, materials, etc.)

Evaluation Procedures	Areas in Need of Further Study
Re-evaluation Date _____	Team Review Date _____

177

suitable placement be sought in the least restrictive environment. A wide range of creative placements and combinations have been used by school systems to serve THI students. The range of possible placements is identified in Table 29.

The cognitive, behavioral, physical, and social vulnerabilities of THI students often make them targets of misperception and susceptible to risk-taking behavior and dares. School peers should be made

TABLE 29

RANGE OF PLACEMENTS USED TO SERVE THI STUDENTS

- **Regular Education** (full day, no provisions)
- **Regular Education** (full day)
  - —former grade repeated
  - —supplemented by after-school tutor
  - —with remedial classes
  - —with summer school
  - —with personal aide
  - —multiple provisions
- **Modified** (full day)
  - —less demanding course load
  - —in-school tutoring
  - —monitored by guidance counselor or consultant
  - —multiple provisions
- **Collapsed** (part day)
  - —one period to 1 half day with regular and/or resource teacher(s)
  - —multiple provisions
- **Special Education**
  - —regular classes with special education consultant
  - —resource services plus monitored regular classes
  - —self-contained
  - —self-contained in separate location or building annex
- **Homebound**
  - —one or several periods at school plus half day homebound
  - —total homebound
- **Eclectic**
  - —combination of part public school services (special ed. and/or regular ed.), homebound services, community-based training, and related services (from school, private therapist, and/or hospital)
- **Residential**
  - —schools
  - —hospitals
  - —institutions

aware of their classmate's condition and the effects of THI (Savage & Carter, 1984). As they demonstrate readiness, classmates should be informed of specific ways to facilitate the recovery process in a manner that is productive and sensitive to both parties.

Rosen and Gerring (1986), in an informal survey of parents of THI school-aged victims, identified a number of common frustrations parents experience during the process of school reintegration: (a) lack of teacher understanding, (b) uncooperative and insensitive regular education teachers, (c) stress and strain from working with their child on homework, (d) parental isolation, (e) the frustration of inappropriate class placements, and (f) the social isolation of their child. This insight into the impressions of parents who have struggled through the process of reintegration underscores the importance of careful preliminary planning and the value of a well-prepared and knowledgeable staff.

Special Placement Decisions

Now that traumatic brain injury has been recognized as one of 13 educational disabilities (Federal Register, 1991), professional education teams are required to provide brain-injured students with an appropriate educational program and procedural safeguards. Educational teams must ensure that the unique needs of THI students are adequately met and that program philosophy and instructional strategies reflect the state of the art. With categorical special education a reality, students must be "educationally diagnosed" before they can qualify for services. It is also a reality that some THI students will continue to be placed in less than appropriate classrooms even though such placement may do them more harm than good (Rosen & Gerring, 1986). A least tantamount in importance to placement is the issue of program integrity and quality of intervention. Placement aside, the educational program should be flexible enough to allow for the frequent modification of program intent and instructional foci. Key educators, administrators, and support staff involved in the program should be knowledgeable about THI and the profile of the returning student. All staff involved should work together to ensure that instructional methods, goals of treatment, methods of evaluation, behavioral management, and underlying philosophy reflect the research and methodology pertinent to traumatic brain injury.

THI students with mild residua who do not qualify for special education or who are presumed recovered on the basis of little more than physical impressions are unlikely to receive transitional or preventative backup without the insistence of an informed advocate. All too often, underestimated yet potentially amenable social, behavioral, and academic deficits escalate into full-blown placement issues. When a traumatically brain-injured student is not found eligible for services under the Individuals with Disabilities Education Act, the requirements of Section 504 of the Rehabilitation Act of 1973 and its implementing regulation may be applicable. Section 504 prohibits discrimination on the basis of handicap by recipients of Federal funds. Because Section 504 is a civil rights law and not a funding law, its requirements are framed in terms different from those of Part B of the IDEA. Section 504 is written in more general terms, hence, by nature, its protections extend to some who do not meet the eligibility requirements as they are specified in Part B. Section 504 requires that all elementary and secondary education programs receiving Federal funds address the needs of children who are considered "handicapped." A handicapped person is defined as any person who has a physical or mental impairment which substantially limits a major life function. Learning, walking, and talking are considered examples of major life functions. Under Section 504, a local education agency must provide a free, appropriate public education to qualified handicapped children. A free, appropriate public education, under Section 504, consists of regular or special education and related aids and services designed to meet individual needs in accordance with the regulatory requirements on educational setting, evaluation, placement, and procedural safeguards. Education must be provided in a regular education classroom unless it can be demonstrated that education in the regular classroom with the use of supplementary aids and services cannot be achieved satisfactorily (34 CFR 104.34). Many school divisions follow the same procedures described in Part B of IDEA to ensure the protections required in Section 504.

Certainly, not all THI students will require special education services in order to benefit from their educational experience. Furthermore, the irregular ability profiles that often emerge following THI, along with the characteristic potential of THI students to recapture lost functions, will more than likely justify at least partial integration opportunities for a number of THI students by the time they graduate. Hence, regular educators should be equally prepared to address the needs of the THI. A range of strategies suitable for regular education classrooms is offered in Table 30.

Because of the nature of their condition, THI students on the whole will require more frequent evaluations, program revisions, and support services; more organized methods of behavioral management; a stronger emphasis upon relearning; and the provision of such process-oriented services as memory therapy and language and perceptual retraining (Begali, 1987; Cohen et al., 1985; Levin et al., 1983; Molnar et al., 1983; NHIF, 1985; Rosen & Gerring, 1986). Community resources

TABLE 30

STRATEGIES FOR REGULAR EDUCATORS SERVING THE TRAUMATICALLY
BRAIN-INJURED STUDENT

- arrange for preferential seating
- use small group instruction
- increase structure and predictability of learning environment
- increase response time
- repeat and simplify verbal instructions
- pair verbal instructions with visual cues
- minimize distractions
- impose individualized behavioral management system
- chart daily progress
- modify test delivery
- provide peer tutors
- require memory log (to record facts often forgotten)
- highlight key points in content reading
- shorten school day or reduce course load
- communicate with child's other teachers
- assign a note taker
- solicit consultation from "expert" in TBI
- seek services of resource teacher
- use self-paced instruction or computer-assisted learning
- provide word processor and computer access
- offer use of suitable software programs
- permit use of calculators and tape recorders
- reduce complicated tasks into smaller steps
- refer for vocational assessment and training
- refer for counseling services
- maintain contact with parents
- redirect inappropriate behavior

---

should be sought to supplement the services of the public school as needed. When an appropriate program cannot be developed from school and local resources, it may be necessary to contract the services of a within-state school system or consider alternative residential placement. The NHIF has published a national directory of head injury rehabilitation programs and facilities (see Appendix A).

Case Illustration

A 16-year-old (S.R.) of High Average to Superior intelligence sustained a severe closed head injury as a result of a horseback riding incident. Upon arrival in the emergency room, the patient showed decerebrate rigidity, was unresponsive to visual, auditory, and verbal stimuli, and was in a state of recurrent convulsive seizures (*status epilepticus*). The initial Glasgow Coma Scale score was 3. Serial CT scans revealed posttraumatic cortical atrophy (more prominent on the left). Secondary complications included severe hypoxia, diffuse cerebral edema, elevated intracranial pressure (ICP), slight brain shifting, and mild enlargement of the third and lateral ventricles. The prognosis for survival at this point was extremely poor. After 1 month of intensive care, however, S.R. was transferred to a rehabilitation center for a rigorous interdisciplinary treatment program aimed at maximizing recovery. (Table 31 shows the long-term treatment plàn and services provided over a 4-year period.) Within 2 months, the patient was able to ambulate with major assistance and was taking feedings via gastrostomy tube. Within 1 year of the injury, S.R. was capable of independent ambulation and minimal self-care. Small but steady gains had been made with respect to receptive language, short-term memory, attention and concentration, visual-motor coordination, and visual discrimination. From a developmental perspective, S.R.'s cognitive skills ranged from 1 month (speech) to 6 years (visual recognition, visual memory, visual discrimination). At 2 years post trauma, local school personnel, rehabilitative staff, and family met to devise an eclectic service plan for S.R. made up of continued outpatient therapy from a local hospital and rehabilitation center and public school services. S.R.'s cognitive abilities at this juncture (chronological age = 18 years) ranged between 4 months (speech) and 7 years (visual and tactile perception). At 3 years post trauma, global aphasia, intellectual loss (with severe retrograde amnesia and short-term memory impairment), and apraxia remained the most disabling and profound residua. Although capable of understanding verbal language when combined with gesture at a level comparable to that of the average 3-year-old, with the exception of several incomprehensible sounds, S.R. remained essentially nonverbal. Selective use of gesture and facial expresson to communicate was beginning to emerge and estimated at about 12 months developmentally. Impulsive behavior and unpredictable tendencies, an inability to judge environmental hazards, and physical and cognitive dependency made continuous supervision at home and school mandatory.

The diffuse damage produced by the trauma and widespread cerebral derangement that followed made a developmental approach to rehabilitation particularly well suited in this case. S.R.'s age, however, required that environmentally based functional training and compensation be incorporated as well. In an effort to stimulate as many neuronal pathways as possible, S.R.'s treatment program was designed to tax as many different regions of the brain as possible. Deliberate attempts were made to include tasks that stimulated the involvement of cortical (higher level) as well as sub-cortical (lower level, cerebellar) functions; left- and right-hemisphere functions; anterior (motor) and posterior (sensory) functions; frontal, temporal, parietal, and occipital lobes; and psychomotor, cognitive, and affective domains. Toward these major goals, specific strategies were combined to form a continuum of both active and passive stimulation activities and direct skill redevelopment training. S.R.'s program included: developmental, functional, and adaptive components, auditory, visual, tactile, proprioceptive, and kinesthetic activities; cross-modality (integrative) objectives; word-symbol (linguistic) and visual-spatial (nonlinguistic) activities; familiar and unfamiliar stimuli; requirements for memory-based problem solving as well as trial and error experimentation; and structured and unstructured tasks.

Regular assessment was conducted and probes for the resolution of higher level functions were routinely taken to chart progress and to "test" for preserved engrams. In spite of significant cortical atrophy and diffuse cerebral involvement, diminished cognitive capacity, and expressive and receptive language deficits, it was determined that S.R. had retained the ability to recognize selected printed words, and learn new ones (as demonstrated by matching, pointing, and facial expressions), because of relatively well-preserved visual discrimination and visual memory skills.

A number of the important elements of optimal programming for school-aged survivors of THI are exemplified in the aforementioned

TABLE 31

LONG-TERM TREATMENT PLAN FOR SEVERELY THI ADOLESCENT (CASE EXAMPLE)

Program Site	Duration	GCS[a]	Level of Cognitive Functioning[b] GOS[c]	Therapy/ Services	Treatment Strategies/Procedures
A. Emergency Room Operating Room	1 day	3	I	Neurosurgery Radiology	Endotracheal intubation and ventilator; ICP pressure monitor; CT scan; EEG; X-rays, anti-convulsant therapy (Dilantin, Valium, Phenobarbitol)
Surgical Intensive Care Unit (SICU)	1 day				
B. Pediatric Intensive Care Unit (PICU)	17 days	4	II	Pediatric medicine/ Nursing Neurosurgery Orthopedics Physical Therapy (PT) Occupational Therapy (OT)	EEG; CT scan; nasogastric tube; ICP pressure monitor removed; treated for edema and pneumonia, medications adjusted; monitoring of vital signs, fluids, etc.; short arm cast for dislocated wrist; passive range-of-motion exercises, sensory stimulation
Neurosurgical Unit	10 days				
C. Pediatric rehabilitation center	11 mos.	10	III-IV (SD)	Pediatric medicine/Nursing PT/OT Recreational Therapy (RT) Speech/Language Therapy (SLT) Special Education Social Work (SW) Psychology Neurosurgery	CT scan, EEG, Phenobarbitol, gastrostomy, Tegretol (at 7 mos.); wheelchair positioning, activities of daily living (ADL), toilet training, balance and mobilization retraining, hydrotherapy; oral stimulation, language stimulation, sensory stimulation and integration training; developmentally based cognitive retraining, computer activities; family counseling, psychological/ neuropsychological assessment, weekly interdisciplinary team meetings with family participation

(continued)

TABLE 31
(CONTINUED)

Program Site	Duration	GCS[a]	Level of Cognitive Functioning[b] GOS[c]	Therapy/ Services		Treatment Strategies/Procedures
D. Transitional program (Outpatient therapy at local hospital and rehab center)	10 mos.	—	IV-V (SD)	Outpatient: (hrs. per week)		Sensory integration (systematic tactile, vestibular, olfactory, auditory, visual input and stimulation); video and computer activities, developmentally based instruction, visual-motor retraining, language stimulation training, visual communication training, hydrotherapy, recreational activities, ADL, toilet training; community-based instruction, family counseling, psychological and neuropsychological assessment, medical follow-up, monthly team meeting with parent participation
				PT	(3)	
				OT	(4)	
				RT	(1)	
				SLT	(5)	
				Cognitive retraining	(2)	
				Special education	(2)	
				Psychology	(1)	
				Pediatric medicine	(1)	
E. Outpatient/Public school	12 mos.	—	V-VI (SD)	Outpatient:		Sensory integration, cognitive retraining, visual communication training, developmentally based individualized instruction, community-based instruction; ADL, toilet training, recreational therapy; family counseling, shunt placed for hydrocephalus, team meetings with parent participation
				PT	(3)	
				OT	(3)	
				RT	(1)	
				SLT	(3)	
				Psychology	(1)	
				Pediatric medicine	(1)	
				Special education	(14)	
				Neurosurgery		

(continued)

185

TABLE 31
(CONTINUED)

Program Site	Duration	GCS[a]	Level of Cognitive Functioning[b] GOS[c]	Therapy/Services	Treatment Strategies/Procedures
F. Public School/Outpatient	Continued through year of 22 birthday	—	V-VI (SD)	Special education Outpatient: PT OT SLT Psychology	(27) Cognitive retraining, language stimulation, developmentally based instruction, computer activities, (3) community-based instruction, toilet training, sensory (2) and bilateral coordination training, family counseling, (3) medical monitoring, team meetings with parent (1) participation

Note. [a]Glasgow Coma Scale used only to describe early stages of recovery.
[b]Rancho Los Amigos Level of Cognitive Functioning used to illustrate progress over time.
[c]Glasgow Outcome Scale (SD = Severely Disabled)

case. It is necessary to point out, however, that the comprehensiveness of this treatment plan was due in main part to (a) the receptiveness and availability of appropriate local resources and well-trained specialists, (b) the commitment of the family and their active participation in all phases of treatment, and (c) the patient's ability to adapt to various treatment regimens and everchanging routines. The inclusion of this case example is not meant to suggest that all treatment programs must incorporate the same strategies to the same degree. The suitability of a treatment program following THI is best measured by (a) the ability of its facilitators to respond with knowledge and sensitivity to the nature of the injury; (b) the client's age, residual skills, and pattern of dysfunction; and (c) the realities of the family system and its long-term plans for placement. Educational treatment programs for THI must be responsive to the unique needs of the student in ways that reflect the research and methodology pertinent to THI.

Toward Quality Educational Service Delivery for THI Students

Without a sense of direction, efforts to promote the educational success and continued progress of THI children and adolescents are easily diluted. Educational programs for THI students should ensure that professional training and expertise, instructional methods, and program practices parallel the state of the art in head injury rehabilitation. Because no two injuries manifest the same neurobehavioral consequences, rate, pattern, or degree of recovery, educational programs for the THI child need to be responsive and timely. A quality program is one that is organized to permit the mobilization of resources in ways that facilitate (a) home–school coordination, (b) effective hospital-to-school transitions, (c) multidisciplinary collaboration, (d) environmental control, (e) low pupil–teacher ratio, (f) individualized and intensive instructional techniques, (g) an emphasis on process-specific approaches, and (h) adoption of state-of-the-art practices.

Home–School Coordination. Brain injury can adversely affect behavioral, psychological, social, and academic performances. Memory, attention, information processing, interpersonal relations, self-perception, and judgment can be impaired as a result. Coordination and consistency help counteract the neurobehavioral effects of THI. When the rules and expectations for behavior at home run contrary to those at school or when supervision is sporadically applied, behaviors are subject to decline and disorder. As a result, potentially surmountable problems can markedly escalate. School personnel will need to involve parents in preliminary planning meetings for returning students. Regular phone calls, progress reports, and team meetings should become part of a routine that ensures thorough communication, rehabilitative continuity, and, ultimately, the continued progress of THI students upon school re-entry.

Effective Transitioning. It is not uncommon for children with severe injuries to be served in a hospital or rehabilitation center for less than 1 year and by the school system for as many as 12 to 15 years. Although the medical and educational systems represent two adjacent segments of the treatment continuum, each operates under different state and federal mandates, answers to different local governing boards, and, with regard to immediate and long-range goals, has different treatment constraints. Ethical codes, customs, and practicality further dictate precise modes of operation and program objectives. An appreciation for alternate service delivery models by those involved will ease the transition process. When treatment responsibilities are transferred from an acute care facility to the public school, careful planning and coordination are needed to minimize the effects of organizational differences. As is typically the case, transfers from a medical facility to the public school take place during a highly critical stage of recovery and period of rapid change; the need for interagency coordination and advanced preparation becomes all the more imperative. The principal goal of transition from one model or segment of the continuum to another, whether it be from the medical facility to school or from school to the community, should be to ensure that the medical, psychological, educational, social, and vocational needs of the THI child are thoroughly conveyed and that regression due to transfer is minimized. Short-term adjustment counseling can provide an added measure of support and stability. Regularly scheduled opportunities for the student to discuss specific concerns will minimize problem escalation.

Integrated Support Services and Multidisciplinary Collaboration. Functional impairments following THI are generally the interactive result of several generic deficits upon a situational context. For example, memory problems are easily compounded by attention, concentration, and perceptual deficits and further exacerbated by specific situational demands. When therapeutic interventions are delivered in disjointed fashion, that is, without purpose and continuity, head-injured persons whose ability to process and consolidate varied information is typically impaired will be unable to make sense of the fragmentation. Hence, remedial interventions stand a limited chance of being successfully incorporated into behavioral repertoires (Ben-Yishay & Gold, 1990). Each team member must subscribe to an agreed-upon response to specific behaviors. Bridging techniques such as regularly scheduled treatment plan reviews and progress assessments, the appointment of a case manager, daily progress documentation, home–school coordination, and cooperative goal development promote continuity and enhance program effectiveness. Members of the child's educational treatment team should include teachers, parents, rehabilitative specialists, and community providers.

Environmental Control. Traumatic brain injury will often affect functional abilities. For example, school-aged children who have sustained THI may find it difficult to recall class schedules, locate classes, organize materials, and adjust to variations in teaching styles and routine. Upon initial re-entry, some THI students will require a self-contained placement to allow for systematic observation and the consistent redirection of behavior under controlled conditions (Telzrow, 1987). Allowances will need to be made for the cognitive limitations that inhibit accurate assessment of environmental cues and the production of prosocial responses (Wood, 1990b). Once coping abilities improve, the THI student may be gradually and systematically introduced to the less predictable, more demanding, and normalized facets of the school experience.

Low Pupil–Teacher Ratio. Data on the most successful cognitive rehabilitation programs substantiate the efficacy of a low instructor-to-client ratio (Ben-Yishay, 1980). Not all students will require a small class size. Those whose deficits are severe, however, are likely to benefit from intensive training, close supervision, minimal distractions, and frequent corrective feedback, the likes of which are not easily attained in large classrooms.

Individualized and Intensive Instructional Opportunities. The rapid and unpredictable changes that follow THI require dynamic and responsive approaches. The consequences resulting from brain injury vary dramatically from one individual to another. Most THI students will require frequent probing for recovered functions. Fluctuating performance profiles will warrant frequent programmatic changes and further modification of instructional objectives. Depending upon the age and status of the student, direct retraining and or compensatory strategies may be employed. It is not uncommon for THI students to experience notable problems with memory and new learning, two skills of critical importance in the academic setting. Consequently, THI students will by nature require more practice opportunities, repetition, and time to learn. One way of maximizing instructional time is to limit involvement in nonessential activities. For example, time spent in transitional and extracurricular classes should be limited during the early stages of school re-entry (Telzrow, 1987). THI students in a critical stage of recovery for whom the traditional summer vacation would result in regression such that recoupment within a reasonable period of time would not be possible and for whom self-sufficiency would be significantly jeopardized may qualify for an extended school program (Slenkovich, 1987).

Emphasis on Process. Emphasis should be placed upon progressive, functional, and process-oriented instruction. Such processes as memory, attention, reasoning, and communication are far more important to emphasize than isolated skill deficits. Whether the focus is on language, attention, or academic remediation, instruction conducted during the early stages of recovery should take into account the THI student's preferred style of learning and neuropsychological profile. The rate, amount, duration, and complexity of stimulus input should be adjusted to match cognitive ability. As the student's ability to handle greater demands increases, so should the complexity of cognitive and situational demands increase.

State-of-the-Art Programming. An "appropriate education" is defined by the state of the art in both teacher training and instructional methodology. Federal standards for the education of disabled children are intended to encourage educational systems to adopt effective practices. A THI child's potential to benefit from the school experience is delimited when educational teams lack the knowledge and technical expertise required to promote academic, social, and emotional growth. Children and adolescents who return to school following traumatic brain injury will present unfamiliar challenges to school professionals. More than likely, school policies and procedures will require some adjusting to reflect the standards imposed by IDEA and new trends in head injury rehabilitation. For example,

1. THI children are likely to require instructional modifications, such as an increased emphasis upon process training, a slower intructional pace, regular probing for the return of lost functions, frequent practice and repetition, modality-specific training, a modified approach to behavioral management, concrete language, and predictable routines (Begali, 1987; Blosser & DePompei, 1991).

2. Moderately and severely injured children are likely to require early vocational assessment, rehabilitative counseling, and transition services (a coordinated set of activities designed to promote movement from school to postschool activities, such as vocational training, supported employment, independent living services, etc.) (Federal Register, 1991). A focus on the redevelopment of practical and independent living skills may be required. Basic skills such as using public transportation, money management, shopping, attending public events, preparing a meal, or brushing one's teeth may need to be task-analyzed in order to determine the area of breakdown in preparation for retraining.

3. The neuropsychological consequences of THI require that adjustments be made in the interpretation of formal test results and the ways in which tests are administered.

4. THI children are likely to require an integrated service plan that may include special education and related services such as speech/language therapy, psychological counseling, rehabilitative counseling, occupational therapy, physical therapy, special transportation, specialized equipment, adapted physical education, or a personal assistant.

5. Many THI children will require programmatic adjustments such as a shortened school day, reduced course load, or extended school year. Individualized education plans will need to be revised to reflect changes in student performance and service needs.

There is no guarantee that THI students will be well served simply because one is aware of what is effective, as professionals and systems must successfully incorporate state-of-the-art strategies into an integrated whole. Nonetheless, without an awareness of where to go, how, and why, systems will continue to evolve blindly on the basis of misperception and outdated practices. Meanwhile, the THI student loses precious time and recovery potential.

APPENDIX A

Resources for Educators Working With Traumatically Head-Injured Children

Information & Resource Organizations

American Foundation for the Blind
15 West 16th Street
New York, NY 10011
212-620-2000

American Physical Therapy Association
1111 North Fairfax Street
Alexandria, VA 22314
703-684-2782

American Occupational Therapy Association
1383 Picard Drive, P.O. Box 1735
Rockville, MD 20850
301-948-9626

American Speech, Language & Hearing Association
10801 Rockville Pike
Rockville, MD 20852
301-897-5700

Association for the Advancement of Rehabilitation Technology
101 Connecticut Avenue, N.W., Suite 700
Washington, D.C. 20036
202-857-1199

Center for Special Education Technology
Council for Exceptional Children
1929 Association Drive
Reston, VA 22091
703-620-3600

Epilepsy Foundation of America
4351 Garden City Drive, Suite 406
Landover, MD 20785
301-459-3700

Learning Disability Association of America
4516 Library Road
Pittsburgh, PA 15234
412-341-1515

National Head Injury Foundation
1140 Connecticut Avenue, N.W., Suite 812
Washington, D.C. 20036
800-444-6443

National Rehabilitation Information Center
8455 Colesville Road, Suite 935
Silver Spring, MD 20910-3319
800-346-2742

Adaptive Equipment/Resources

Name:	*Car Door Reacher, Extension Hook*
Manufacturer:	Trujillo Industries 5040 Firestone Boulevard South Gate, CA 90280
Description:	Chrome-plated hook, 18 inches long. Can be used to close car doors or to pull wheelchair into position.
Name:	*Carrying Bag for Walker [or Wheelchair]*
Manufacturer:	Jandor 1028 Taft Road Duluth, MN 55803
Description:	Carrying bag with flapped velcro closure.

Name:	*Emergency Alert Systems "Lifeline"*
Manufacturer:	Lifeline Systems, Inc. One Arsenal Market Place Watertown, MA 02172
Description:	Emergency alert systems rentable by the month. Hand held push button transmitter sends signals to receiver unit attached to telephone. Unit automatically dials hospital and hospital calls back.

Name:	*Encoding Control Switch "Numberboard"*
Manufacturer:	Scitronics, Inc. 523 South Clewell Street Bethlehem, PA 18015
Description:	Numberboard communication device for persons with limited motor control who cannot press keys on a standard keyboard. Digits are entered for desired words or phrases.

Name:	*Large Print Display Processor,* *"Visualtek, Model #DP-11"*
Manufacturer:	Vtek 1625 Olympic Boulevard Santa Monica, CA 90404
Description:	Large print display processor. Compatible with IBM PC or PC/XT. Enlarges standard dot matrix video display into clear solid magnified characters up to 16X their original size.

Name:	*Multilingual and Symbolic Language Systems* *"Talking Pictures Sticker Kit"*
Manufacturer:	Crestwood Company 6625 North Sidney Place Milwaukee, WI 53209
Description:	Pressure sensitive stickers which demonstrate survival needs; reusable.

Name: *Pill Organizer, "Mediplanner"*

Manufacturer: Apex Medical Corp.
                      807 West 106th Street
                      Bloomington, MN 55420
                            or
                      Local Pharmacy

Description: Holds pills for 7 days with four compartments per day. Twenty-eight compartments open individually for "morning," "noonday," "evening," and "bedtime."

Name: *Speech Synthesizer/Voice Output Module*

Manufacturer: Sensory Interface Equipment
                      4442 Kasson Road
                      Syracuse, NY 13215

Description: Digital displays are converted to synthesized speech.

Name: *Voice Output Word Processor Program*
                      "Talking SC Word Processor"

Manufacturer: Micro Talk
                      337 South Peterson Avenue
                      Louisville, KY 40206

Description: Talking word processor program for voice output computer. Requires Apple II, Apple IIe, or Apple IIc and ECHO Speech Synthesizer.

Name: *"Wizard" Microcomputer*

Manufacturer: Commercially available where electronic equipment is sold (e.g., Radio Shack)

Description: Hand-held microcomputer with timeclock and calendar that allows the user to enter important events such as social appointments, class or therapy schedules, and medication regimens. An audible alarm chimes at designated time. Includes address book, telephone directory, and calendar. Can drive its own printer and is compatible with desktop computer.

196

Appendix A

Cognitive Rehabilitation: Selected Bibliography and Annotation

Adamovich, B. B., Henderson, J. A., & Auerbach, S. (1985). *Cognitive rehabilitation of closed head injured patients: A dynamic approach.* San Diego, CA: College-Hill Press.

Overview of the literature to date on cognitive rehabilitation. The authors break down theories of cognitive rehabilitation into information processing, cognitive, and neurophysiological components. Includes step-by-step treatment protocols and procedures.

Bach-y-Rita, P. (1981). Central nervous system lesion: Sprouting and unmasking in rehabilitation. *Archives of Physical Medicine and Rehabilitation, 62,* 413-417.

Stresses that neural plasticity is important in recovery of functional skills. Discusses diaschisis, regenerative sprouting, collateral sprouting, and unmasking (functional compensation). Factors influencing neuroplasticity include time course of recovery, delay of intervention, age, environmental factors, motivation, and neuropharmacology.

Bagnato, S. J., Mayes, S. D., Nichter, C. & Domoto, V. (1988). An interdisciplinary neurodevelopmental assessment model for brain-injured infants and preschool children. *Journal of Head Trauma Rehabilitation, 3*(2), 75-86.

Describes the design, content, and use of an interdisciplinary system to plan early childhood treatment for brain injuries (INSPECT). The INSPECT system uses administrative and clinical appraisal and three types of assessment (norm based, adaptive curriculum based, and clinical judgment). The case of a 33-month-old brain-injured girl illustrates how the INSPECT system synchronizes interdisciplinary assessment, plans treatment, monitors the effectiveness of interventions, and profiles patient progress.

Barth, J., & Boll, T. (1981). Rehabilitation and treatment of central nervous system dysfunction: A behavioral medicine perspective. In C. Prokop & L. Bradley (Eds.), *Medical psychology: Contributions to behavioral medicine.* New York: Academic Press.

Includes review of cognitive rehabilitation literature. Discusses neuropathology, assessment, factors affecting recovery, and intervention modalities. Emotional factors and coping are emphasized.

Treatment techniques discussed included behavior modification, memory retraining, a team approach to sexual dysfunction, group therapy, biofeedback training, and cognitive retraining.

Ben-Yishay, Y. (1983). Cognitive remediation viewed from the perspective of a systematic clinical research program in rehabilitation. *Cognitive Rehabilitation, 1*(5), 4-6.

General discussion of cognitive remediation. Offers guidelines central to developing remediation strategies. Recovery depends upon the extent of the deficits, the individual's awareness of his or her problem, motivation, and responsiveness to treatment. Discusses importance of integration of training experiences and generalization.

Ben-Yishay, Y., & Diller, L. (1981). Rehabilitation of cognitive and perceptual defects in people with traumatic brain damage. *International Journal of Rehabilitation Research, 4,* 208-210.

Discusses the modular treatment program at New York University. Components include: (1) Orientation Remedial Module, (2) Eye-hand Coordination, (3) Perceptual-cognitive Integration, (4) Visual Information Processing, (5) Verbal, Logical Reasoning, (6) Interpersonal Skills Module, (7) Group Therapy, and (8) Community Activities Component. Thirteen brain-injured individuals underwent 20 weeks of treatment. The areas showing greatest improvement were attention, concentration, and interpersonal skills.

Bolger, J. (1982). Cognitive retraining: A developmental approach. *Clinical Neuropsychology, 4*(2), 66-70.

Discusses an approach which integrates the developmental models, Luria's ideas, and operant principles. It involves three goals: (1) improving mental strategies, (2) reducing task demands, and (3) increasing information capacity. Video tasks, behavioral techniques, group therapy, and tutoring are discussed.

Bracy, O. L. (1982). *Cognitive rehabilitation programs for brain injured and stroke patients* [Computer Programs]. Indianapolis, IN: Psychological Software Services, Inc.

Computer programs for retraining attention, visuospatial skills, memory, and problem-solving skills.

Carter, L. T., Caruso, J. L., Languirand, M. A., & Berard, M. A. (1980). Cognitive skills remediation in stroke and non-stroke elderly. *Clinical Neuropsychology, 2*(3), 109-113.

Study utilizing paper-and-pencil tasks from *The Thinking Skills Workbook* to retrain 37 rehabilitation patients. The patients were matched for type of lesion, age, and pretest scores on the tasks and were randomly assigned to treatment or no-treatment groups. After four weeks of training, experimental patients showed greater improvement on the tasks, particularly on visual-spatial and letter cancellation tasks. The control group, however, performed better on a verbal free-recall task.

Carter, L. T., Caruso, J. L., Languirand, M. A., & Berard, M. A. (1980). *The thinking skills workbook: A cognitive skills remediation manual for adults.* Springfield, IL: Charles C. Thomas.

Paper-and-pencil tasks such as letter cancellation, word recognition, categorization, and basic arithmetic drills which can be used to retrain brain-injured patients.

Craine, J. F. (1982). Principles of cognitive rehabilitation. In L. E. Trexler (Ed.), *Cognitive rehabilitation: Conceptualization and intervention.* New York: Plenum Press.

Outlines eight principles of neurotraining: (1) Plasticity of function within the central nervous system, (2) The dynamic nature of neurological organization, (3) Learning results from repeated activity and is organized into functional systems, (4) Retraining recapitulates developmental stages, (5) Complex higher cortical functions represent integration of sensory modalities, (6) Retraining focuses on the dynamics of learning rather than on specific content, (7) Training should be deficit-specific, and (8) Consistent and direct feedback to patients is essential.

Craine, J. F., & Gudeman, H. E. (1981). *The rehabilitation of brain functions: Principles, procedures, and techniques of neurotraining.* Springfield, IL: Charles C. Thomas.

This is a workbook which includes paper-and-pencil exercises for developing visual-perceptual, visual-motor, and visual-scanning skills, and dexterity.

Crewe, N., & Athlestan, G. (1981). Functional assessment in vocational rehabilitation: A systematic approach to diagnosis and goal setting. *Archives of Physical Medicine and Rehabilitation, 62,* 299-305.

Describes Functional Assessment Inventory (FAI). The scale measures cognitive functioning, motor functioning, personality and social behavior, vocational assessment, medical evaluation, and financial aspects.

Diller, L., Ben-Yishay, Y., Gertsman, L. J., et al. (1974). *Studies in cognition and rehabilitation: Rehabilitation monograph No. 50.* New York: New York University Medical Center, Institute of Rehabilitation Medicine.

One of a series of monographs published by New York University describing the results of the cognitive rehabilitation program at the rehabilitation center.

Diller, L., & Gordon, W. (1981). Interventions for cognitive deficits in brain-injured adults. *Journal of Consulting and Clinical Psychology, 49,* 822-834.

Article reviewing the various treatment modalities for cognitive retraining. Describes modular approach used at NYU which incorporates continuous and immediate feedback, cueing, gradually increasing level of difficulty, and generalization training. Modules address visuospatial skills, psychomotor speech, abstract thinking, attention/vigilance, and social skills.

Engum, E. S., & Lambert, E. W. (1990). Restandardization of the Cognitive Behavioral Driver's Inventory. *Cognitive Rehabilitation, 8*(6), 20-27.

The Cognitive Behavioral Driver's Inventory was administered to 232 rehabilitation patients to include those with traumatic head injury to restandardize the normative tables and increase the rigor and precision of the decision-making process. Normative tables and guidelines provide professionals with an objective means for evaluating the operational driving skills of brain-injured clients.

Gianutsos, R. (1980). What is cognitive rehabilitation? *Journal of Rehabilitation,* July–September, 36-40.

The author defines cognitive rehabilitation as "a service developed to remediate disorders of perception, memory, and language in brain-injured persons."

Gianutsos, R., & Klitzner, C. (1981). *Computer programs for cognitive rehabilitation.* Bayport, NY: Life Sciences Associates.

Computer programs for assessing and retraining perceptual and memory disorders.

Gummow, L., Miller, P., & Dustman, R. E. (1983). Attention and brain injury: A case for cognitive rehabilitation of attentional deficits. *Clinical Psychology Review, 3,* 255-274.

Review of cognitive rehabilitation literature from the perspective of attentional deficits. Discusses the computer as a motivational tool.

Hagen, C. (1988). Treatment of aphasia: A process approach. *Journal of Head Trauma Rehabilitation, 3*(2), 23-33.

Discusses an approach to the treatment of aphasia. The approach is directed toward increasing the efficiency of language processing rather than compensation for language skills. Treatment involves the identification of rehabilitative stimuli that will facilitate processing at the point of breakdown in language processing. Case examples provided.

Heilman, K. M., & Valenstein, E. (Eds.). (1979). *Clinical neuropsychology.* New York: Oxford University Press.

Covers behavioral and intellectual disorders associated with brain dysfunction, such as aphasia, alexia, agraphia, acalculia, body schema disturbances, apraxia, visuospatial disorders, agnosia, neglect, frontal lobe dysfunction, memory problems, and dementia. Recovery and treatment are addressed.

Jurko, M. F. (1981). Recent developments in brain rehabilitation. *Southern Medical Journal, 74*(6), 727-730.

Describes techniques used at NYU for remediating visual-spatial neglect, sensory-spatial problems, higher order reasoning skills, categorical thinking, and recent memory deficits.

Katz, R., & Nagy, V. T. (1984). CATS: Computerized aphasia treatment system. *Cognitive Rehabilitation, 2*(4), 8-11.

Discusses the use of specially designed software for treatment of aphasia.

Knight, R. G., & Wooles, I. M. (1980). Experimental investigation of chronic organic amnesia: A review. *Psychological Bulletin, 88*(3), 753-771.

Review of literature on memory deficits. Supporting evidence on the application of various rehabilitation principles, viz., supply verbal labels for nonverbal material, increase depth of processing, lengthen rehearsal time, extend stimulus exposure time, use organizational cues within stimulus presentation.

Larose, S., Gagnon, S., Ferland, C., & Pepin, M. (1989). Psychology of computers: XIV. Cognitive rehabilitation through computer games. *Perceptual & Motor Skills, 69*(3), 851-858.

Forty boys and girls (aged 8-14 years) with attention problems were matched with controls to test the efficiency of computer programs as a cognitive tool. A 12-hour training program with the game Super Breakout served as the intervention. Experimental subjects showed improvement on scanning and tracking variables.

Lawson, M. J., & Rice, D. N. (1989). Effects of training in the use of executive strategies on a verbal memory problem resulting from closed head injury. *Journal of Clinical and Experimental Neuropsychology, 11*(6), 842-854.

An executive training strategy was employed with a 15-year-old male with closed head injury in an attempt to improve recall performance. Training produced evidence of improvement in paired-associate and free recall tests.

Lynch, W. J. (1983). Cognitive retraining using microcomputer games and commercially available software. *Cognitive Rehabilitation, 1*(1), 19-22.

Application of commercially available video games such as "Pong," "Breakout," and "Brain Games" to retrain attention, concentration, reaction time, and hand-eye coordination in four brain-injured patients. The advantages and disadvantages of video games for cognitive retraining are discussed.

Lynch, W. J. (1984). *A guide to Atari home computer (600XL/800XL/ 1200XL) and Apple II + IIe programs for rehabilitation settings:* 6th edition. Unpublished manuscript. Palo Alto Veterans Administration Medical Center, Brain Rehabilitation Unit, Palo Alto, CA.

Reference describing the commercially available video games and specially designed software for working wth brain-injured patients. Contains practical information for utilizing computer programs in cognitive rehabilitation therapy.

Parente, F. J., & Anderson, J. K. (1983). Techniques for improving cognitive rehabilitation: Teaching organization and encoding skills. *Cognitive Rehabilitation, 1*(4), 20-22.

Computerized memory exercises were used to enhance organizational and encoding abilities in two patients with memory deficits. Training lasted six months and incorporated categorization, chunking, verbal mediation, and mnemonics. Significant increments in memory quotients were noted.

Pollak, I. W., Kohn, H., & Miller, M. H. (1984). Rehabilitation of cognitive function in brain-damaged persons. *The Journal of the Medical Society of New Jersey, 81*(4), 311-315.

An outcome evaluation of cognitive rehabilitation programs at the Rutgers Medical School in Piscataway, N.J. The program utilized a 4-step series of exercises emphasizing (1) the ability to focus and sustain attention, (2) increased capacity and the ability to sequence and categorize information, (3) development of problem-solving strategies, and (4) communication skills. Authors report gains in Performance IQs after 13 weeks of training.

Pollens, R., McBratnie, B. P., & Burton, P. L. (1988). Beyond cognition: Executive function in closed head injury. *Cognitive Rehabilitation, 6*(5), 26-32.

Discusses the relationship between specific skills acquisition and successful community reintegration. Executive function skills include awareness, goal setting, planning, self-initiation, self-monitoring, ability to change set, and strategic behavior. Case descriptions illustrate the effects of these deficits upon the individual, family, and therapeutic process.

Savir, H., Michaelson, I., David, C., Mendelson, L., & Najenson, T. (1977). Homonymous hemianopsia and rehabilitation in fifteen cases of cranio-cerebral injuries. *Scandinavian Journal of Rehabilitation Medicine, 9,* 151-153.

The program at New York University for remediating visual field deficits is discussed. Correlational study examining hemianopsia, dexterity, visual-motor organization, intellectual functions, and rehabilitation outcome. Eleven out of 15 cases with poor rehabilitation outcome showed left hemianopsia and all had some impairment of perceptual motor functions.

Sbordone, R. J. (1983). *Computer programs for neuropsychological testing and cognitive rehabilitation* [Computer Programs]. Foundation Valley, CA: Robert J. Sbordone, PhD, Inc.

Computer programs for testing and retraining memory, attention, and problem-solving skills.

Sena, D. A. (1984). *The effectiveness of cognitive retraining for brain-impaired individuals.* Paper presented at the 92nd Annual Convention of the American Psychological Association, Toronto, Canada.

A combined program of REHABIT (Reitan Evaluation of Hemispheric Abilities and Brain Improvement Training), Atari video-games, specialized software, psychosocial retraining and psychophysiological training was used to treat 12 outpatients. The author noted improvement in 31 of 39 neuropsychological measures after one year of rehabilitation.

Smith, J. (1984). *Microcomputer programs for cognitive rehabilitation.* Dimondale, MI: Hartley Courseware, Inc.

Computer programs developed for use with neurological patients. The structured activities enhance linguistic-cognitive development. Tasks promote categorization, memory, association, and sequencing.

Sohlberg, M. M., & Mateer, C. A. (1989). *Introduction to cognitive rehabilitation: Theory and practice.* New York: Guilford Press.

A highly practical and comprehensive text that provides a solid foundation in basic rehabilitation principles and in-depth reviews of neuropsychological assessment, therapies and research, and specialized techniques for remediating cognitive deficits. Chapters cover such topics as group therapy, the management of psychosocial deficits, and community reintegration.

Weinberg, J., Piasetsky, E., Diller, L., & Gordon, W. (1982). Treating perceptual organization deficits in nonneglecting right brain damaged stroke patients. *Journal of Clinical Neuropsychology, 4,* 59-75.

Visual integration training was used to remediate perceptual deficits in 17 right-hemisphere brain-damaged patients. Eighteen stroke patients serve as "no treatment" controls. The patients in the experimental group showed improvement on 8 out of 12 tests of visuocognitive ability. Controls showed gains on only 1 out of the 12 tests.

Wilson, P. B. (1983). Software selection and use in language and cognitive rehabilitation. *Cognitive Rehabilitation, 1*(1), 9-10.

Author offers suggestions for choosing software to use in remediating brain-injured patients. Software should be flexible, have clear instructions, not be demeaning or juvenile in appearance, provide feedback, vary in level of difficulty, have parameters which can be controlled, be interesting, avoid complex displays, and should present performance data.

Computer Software for Cognitive Rehabilitation

NYU Medical Center
Head Trauma Program
400 East 34th Street, RR119
New York, NY 10017

Computer programs for the THI that address attention/reaction, accuracy, visual discrimination, time estimation, and rhythm synchronization, etc.

Cognitive Educational Software Series
Rehabilitation Programs
353 East State Street
Long Beach, NY 11561

Specialized computer programs which correspond with Rancho Los Amigos' Levels of Cognitive Functioning.

Cognitive Rehabilitation
P.O. Box 29344
Indianapolis, IN 46229

Publication which routinely lists new computer programs for head-injured clients.

A & S Medical Sales, Inc.
723 Franklin Square, Suite 502
Michigan City, IN 46360

Computer software packages that emphasize visual reaction, visual scanning, auditory reaction, perception and training, etc.

Compu-tations, Inc.
P.O. Box 502
Troy, MI 48009

Source for early elementary-level software appropriate for THI.

Life Science Associates
One Fenimore Road
Bayport, NY 11705

Emphasis on perception and memory training.

Psychological Software
P.O. Box 29205
Indianapolis, IN 46229

Specially designed microcomputer software assortment for THI individuals.

Instructional Resources

Academic Therapy Publications
20 Commercial Boulevard
Novato, CA 94947

Assorted educational materials.

Agency for Instructional Television
Box A
Bloomington, IN 47401

Source of instructional and mental health video programs.

Barnell Loft, Ltd.
958 Church Street
Baldwin, Long Island, NY 11510

Specific skills series (using the context, locating the answer, following directions, drawing conclusions, detecting the sequence, etc.)

Communication Skill Builders Stimulation Inc.
P.O. Box 42050-F
Tucson, AZ 85733

Thematic language materials for aphasics.

DLM Inc.
P.O. Box 4500
Allen, TX 75002

Independent living sequential cards, consumer sequential cards, open sequence cards, etc.

Grune & Stratton, Inc.
111 Fifth Avenue
New York, NY 10003

Assorted instructional materials.

Innovative Sciences, Inc.
300 Broad Street
Stamford, CT 06901

Language-based problem solving, analytic thinking, etc.

Institute of Rehabilitation Medicine
NYU Medical Center
400 East 34th Street
New York, NY 10016

Educational approaches to the remediation of cognitive deficits following THI.

Interstate Printers and Publishers, Inc.
19 North Jackson Street
Danville, IL 61832

Source of speech/language rehabilitation workbooks.

Laurel Designs
5 Laurel Avenue, T-65
Belvedere, CA 94920

Cookbook of more than 600 recipes. Easy to follow; contain only four ingredients each.

Lingui Systems, Inc.
Suite 806, 1630 Fifth Avenue
Moline, IL 61265

Manual of exercises for expressive reasoning.

Mason Media, Inc.
Box C
Mason, MI 48854

Source for training film package "Influencing Human Interaction" which describes the use of Interpersonal Process Recall.

Modern Education Corporation
P.O. Box 721
Tulsa, OK 74101

Cognitive and perceptual development workbooks.

National Institute of Mental Health
5600 Fishers Lane
Rockville, MD 20852

Provides catalog of audiovisuals on various mental health topics.

Rifton Equipment for People with Disabilities
Rte. 213
P.O. Box 901
Rifton, NY 12471-0901

Accessories and mobility equipment for disabled persons.

SOI Institute
343 Richmond Street
El Segundo, CA 90245

Assorted instructional materials on reasoning, memory, and cognition.

Wayne State University Press
Detroit, MI 48202

Source for *Brubaker Workbook for Aphasia*. Includes exercises on antonyms; homonyms; syllogisms; what, when, where, why, how questions, etc.

First Aid in Seizure Care

I. Generalized Epilepsy

    A. *Tonic Clonic* (grand mal, major motor)

       The most dramatic kind of seizure activity. Begins with sudden loss of consciousness followed by whole body jerking and rigidity. Generally lasts between 2–3 minutes. Followed by confusion or deep sleep.

STEPS

    1. Help person lie down.
    2. Remove sharp and dangerous objects.
    3. Remove glasses, loosen tight clothing such as belt or tie.
    4. *Do not* try to restrain moving arms or legs (you cannot stop the seizure).
    5. *Do not* force anything between clamped teeth.
    6. *Do not* insert fingers, pens, or pencils into the mouth.

AFTER THE SEIZURE

    1. Turn the person's head to the side to let saliva drain from the mouth.
    2. Let person rest for a short period of time.
    3. Do not give food or drink until fully awake.
    4. It is usually not necessary to call an ambulance unless:
       (a) person does not start breathing;
       (b) person has one seizure after another;
       (c) person requests an ambulance.

B. *Absence* (petit mal)

Begins suddenly. Ongoing activity will cease followed by a blank stare and possibly a brief upward rotation of the eyes or head and mild muscle twitching. Generally lasts between 5–45 seconds. May recur many times a day. Usually requires no emergency steps.

II. Partial Epilepsy

A. *Complex partial* (psychomotor)

Consciousness is lost. Can progress to generalized convulsion. Often accompanied by automatisms (repetitive, purposeless motions). May last between 1 minute to several hours. Confusion generally follows.

STEPS

1. Help person lie down.
2. Remove dangerous obstacles.
3. *Do not* try to restrain or inhibit.
4. Monitor until alert.

B. *Simple partial*

No impairment of consciousness. May involve localized convulsions and posturing. No post-seizure symptoms.

FOR ALL SEIZURE TYPES:

1. Stay CALM. Let the seizure run its course.
2. Preserve person's dignity. Disperse onlookers.
3. Note a description of the seizure activity.
4. Record time seizure began and ended.
5. Let person go on with regular activities once rested and alert.

Sources:

Bagby, G. (1991, Winter). Advances in anticonvulsant therapy. *Headlines*, 2-5, 7-8.

Cereghino, J. J. (1990). Treatment implications from classification of seizures and the epilepsies. In D. B. Smith (Ed.), *Epilepsy: Current approaches to diagnosis and treatment* (pp. 1-25). New York: Raven Press.

University of Virginia Medical Center. (1988). *First aid in seizure care.* Available from Blue Ridge Hospital, Epilepsy Unit, 1 West, Charlottesville, VA 22901.

GLOSSARY

action potential: the brief electrical impulse by which information is conducted along an axon

adventitious: of or pertaining to an accidental condition; not congenital

agnosia: partial or complete inability to recognize sensory stimuli; perception without meaning

ambulatory: able to walk

angiography: radiographic (X-ray) techique capable of visualizing blood vessels following the intravenous injection of a contrast medium

angular gyrus: a convolution in the parietal lobe important in language functions and intersensory processing

anomia: difficulty in finding words, especially those naming objects

anopsia: blindness; loss of both visual fields

anosmia: loss of the sense of smell

anoxia: an abnormal condition characterized by a relative or total lack of oxygen

anterior: of or pertaining to the front

anterograde amnesia: inability to remember events subsequent to head injury

anterograde memory: memory of the moment of injury and the events that follow

aphasia: defect or loss of power of expression by speech, writing, or signs, or of comprehending spoken or written language

apnea: an absence of spontaneous respiration

apraxia: impairment in the ability to perform purposeful acts or to manipulate objects in the absence of paralysis or paresis

ataxia: a disturbance in the coordination of the muscular movements

axon: a thin neuronal process that transmits action potentials away from the cell body to other neurons

basal ganglia: the islands of gray matter within each cerebral hemisphere composed of the putamen, caudate, and globus pallidus. The structure is involved in modulating and modifying motor movements. Damage to the basal ganglia results in involuntary motor movements and disturbances in muscle tone.

baseline: pretreatment behavior; a level of performance upon which the effects of experimental treatments can be assessed

bilateral: occurring on or applying to both sides of the body

Broca's aphasia: an expressive or nonfluent aphasia that results from a lesion to Broca's area of the brain

cerebrospinal fluid (CSF): a clear colorless solution of sodium chloride and other salts which cushions the brain. CSF flows beneath the arachnoid layer in the subarachnoid space

coma: a state of profound unconsciousness

concussion: brief loss of consciousness following a blow to the head

confabulation: the fabrication of experiences recounted to fill in and cover up gaps in memory

contralateral: pertaining to the side of the body opposite the reference point

contusion: a vascular injury resulting in bruising, edema, and the hemorrhage of capillaries

corpus callosum: the band of commissural fibers which connects the two hemispheres and allows for rapid and effective inter-hemisphere communication

cortex: the outer convoluted surface of the brain that is composed of nerve cell bodies and their synaptic connections. It is the highest and most complexly organized center of the brain. The cortex is typically divided into four main lobes: frontal, temporal, parietal, and occipital.

cranial nerves: twelve nerves that originate in the brain stem and control smell, hearing, vision, eye movement, facial sensations, taste, swallowing, and movement of face, neck, shoulder, and tongue muscles

CT scan: computed tomography. An X-ray procedure that provides a three-dimensional reconstruction of brain architecture by way of computer. By varying the angles of the X-ray beam, numerous "slices" of brain tissue can be visualized and distinguished according to the densities of their components

debridement: the removal of dirt, foreign objects, and damaged tissue from a wound in order to prevent infection and promote healing

decussation: the crossing of pathways from one side of the brain to the other

dendrites: the treelike fibers of a neuron that reach toward other nerve cells

diaschisis: a concept introduced by Von Monakow that pertains to the "neural shock" or "functional standstill" experienced by intact areas of the brain as a result of damage to other remote areas

diencephalon: consists of the hypothalamus, thalamus, metathalamus, and the epithalamus of the brain along with most of the third ventricle. This structure is involved in the transmission of information regarding sensation and movement, and exercises control over the endocrine system

diplopia: double vision; perception of two images from a single object

dorsal: toward the back

dysarthria: difficulty in speech production caused by the incoordination of speech apparatus

dyscalculia: an impairment of the ability to perform arithmetical operations

dysgraphia: an impairment of the ability to write

dyslexia: an impairment of the ability to read

dyspraxia: a partial loss of the ability to perform skilled, coordinated movements in the absence of any associated defect in motor or sensory functions

edema: the abnormal accumulation of fluid; swelling resulting from an excessive accumulation of fluid from the blood capillaries which consists of a clear liquid portion of the blood

electroencephalogram (EEG): a graphic chart on which is traced the electrical potential produced by brain cells, as detected by electrodes placed on the scalp. The resulting brain waves are called alpha, beta, delta, and theta rhythms according to the frequencies they produce. Variations in brain-wave activity correlate with neurological conditions, level of consciousness, and psychological states. The EEG is commonly used to detect seizure activity, brain stem disorders; focal lesions, and impaired consciousness. Abnormality is detected on the basis of excessively slow or fast activity and certain spike wave patterns. The EEG is a poor estimate of extent of brain damage and an inaccurate predictor of outcome.

electrolyte balance: the equilibrium between electrolytes in the body. Proper quantities of principal electrolytes and balance among them are necessary for normal function and metabolism.

embolism: the sudden blocking of an artery or vein by a blood clot, bubble of air, deposit of oil or fat, or small mass of cells deposited by the blood current

endotracheal tube: a large-bore catheter inserted through the mouth or nose into the trachea (windpipe). It is used to deliver oxygen, control breathing, and prevent foreign material from entering the lungs

epidural: outside the dura mater

epilepsy: a group of neurological disorders characterized by recurrent episodes of convulsive seizures, abnormal behavior, loss of consciousness, sensory disturbances, or all of the above. An uncontrolled electrical discharge from the nerve cells of the cerebral cortex is common to all forms of epilepsy. *Status epilepticus* is characterized by continual attacks of convulsive seizures which occur without intervals of consciousness. Because irreversible brain damage can result if seizures go unarrested, status epilepticus is considered a medical emergency.

equipotential: pertaining to the theory of brain function which states that while sensory input may be localized, perception and other more complex and higher level processes involve the whole brain. Specific regions of the brain are believed to assume the same functional capabilities and participate on an equal basis with no specialization per se. Accordingly, the effects of brain lesions depend not upon their location, but upon their extent.

functional system theory: modern theory of brain function and organization based on the premise that the cortex consists of a complex integrated hierarchy of functional zones which work together to account for complex forms of behavior. Intact systems can be identified so that areas of lost functions can be bypassed, strengthened, or compensated.

gastrostomy: surgical creation of an artifical opening in the stomach through the abdomen for the purpose of feeding by way of tube

Glasgow Coma Scale (GCS): a quick, practical, and standardized system for assessing degree of conscious impairment and predicting outcome following traumatic head injury

Glasgow Outcome Scale (GOS): a reliable scale for categorizing the outcomes of brain-damaged survivors on the basis of overall social capability (or dependence). The four possible categories of survival are: vegetative state (VS), severe disability (SD), moderate disability (MD), and good recovery (GR).

glial cells: supportive cells of the central nervous system

gray matter: any brain area composed predominantly of cell bodies

gustatory: of or pertaining to the sense of taste

hematoma: a collection of escaped blood trapped within an organ (brain). If the space is limited, pressure slows and may eventually stop the flow or the blood may clot and harden and cause infection.

hemianopsia: a loss of half of visual field

hemiparesis: muscular weakness affecting one side of the body

hemiplegia: paralysis of one side of the body

hemorrhage: a loss of a large quantity of blood in a short period of time

herniation: a protrusion or shifting of the brain or portion of the brain through an abnormal opening in a membrane or other tissue

homonymous hemianopsia: loss of vision in same-sided visual field of both eyes

hydrocephalus: a pathological condition characterized by an abnormal accumulation of cerebrospinal fluid (CSF) and subsequent increase in size of the ventricles. Interference with the normal flow of CSF may be due to an increase in the flow of the fluid, or obstruction (noncommunicating hydrocephalus), or poor reabsorption from the subarachnoid space (communicating hydrocephalus).

hyperphagia: voracious food-seeking behavior and overeating that can occur following THI as a result of damage to the hypothalamus or as a result of disinhibition

hyperthermia: a higher than normal body temperature

hyperventilation: a pulmonary ventilation rate which exceeds that which is metabolically necessary for respiration. It is the result of an increased frequency of breathing due to such complications as asthma, fever, infections, injury to the central nervous system, drugs, and hormones.

hypothalamus: a portion of the diencephalon of the brain. It forms the floor and part of the lateral wall of the third ventricle. It activates, controls, and integrates the peripheral autonomic nervous system, endocrine processes, and functions such as body temperature, sleep, and appetite.

hypotonicity: low muscle tone which occurs primarily in the trunk, but is also seen in the extremities

hypoxia: an inadequate reduced tension of arterial oxygen which results in increased heart and respiratory rates. Breathing failure and coma can ensue in severe cases. Treatment may include oxygen therapy, mechanical ventilation, frequent analysis of blood gases, or respiratory stimulant drugs

incontinence: the inability to control urination or defecation. Urinary incontinence can be caused by aging, infection, lesions in the brain, or bladder damage.

infarct: an area of dead or dying tissue resulting from an obstruction of the blood vessels normally supplying the region

inferior: situated below or lower than the given point of reference

intensive care unit (ICU): a hospital unit in which patients requiring close monitoring receive constant, complex, and detailed health care by specially trained providers

intracranial pressure (ICP): the exertion of force within the brain by intracellular and extracellular fluids capable of causing distortion or displacement of cerebral structures or a reduction of cerebral blood flow. Because the skull is a rigid container of brain tissue, blood, and cerebrospinal fluid, an increased volume of one component, unless accompanied by an equal decrease of another, will result in ICP.

intracranial pressure monitor: a tube inserted through the skull into the space outside the brain or into one of the ventricles. The pressure in the head is measured by a transducer connected to the other end of the line. Some ICP monitors are small catheters, others are hollow metal pressure bolts screwed into the skull.

intravenous line: small catheter threaded into a vein used to deliver fluid, nutrients, and medication to the body

intubation: passage of a tube through the mouth or nose or into the trachea to ensure an airway for oxygen or anesthetic gas

ipsilateral: located on the same side of the body as the point of reference

laterality: of or relating to the sides

lesion: any visible local abnormality of the tissues of the body; any damage to the nervous system

localization: the one-to-one correspondence between a specific function and a precise location in the brain. Localization theory implies that all behaviors can be traced to an associated and specific area of the brain.

magnetic resonance imaging (MRI): a diagnostic technique that uses nonionizing forms of enegy to produce sectional images of the human body. A strong magnetic field is used in conjunction with a radio-frequency oscillating magnetic field to stimulate signals from atoms in living tissue. These signals are reconstructed by a computer into sectional images in any plane.

Melodic Intonation Therapy: a specific teaching program which aims to reestablish language in aphasic patients by means of melodic intonation

meninges: any one of three membranes that enclose the brain and spinal cord, comprising the dura mater, pia mater, and arachnoid

morbidity: an abnormal condition of quality

mortality: the condition of being subject to death; rate of death usually expressed per 1,000, 10,000, or 100,000

multimodality evoked potential (MEP): a tracing of brain waves measured on the surface of the head at various places which are elicited by visual, auditory, or somatosensory stimuli

myelin: the lipid substance forming an insulating sheath around certain nerve fibers

myelinization: formation of myelin or axons; used by some as a measure of maturation

nasogastric tube (NG tube): a tube passed into the stomach through the nose. Initially the tube is used to remove gas and secretions from the stomach, later it may be used to instill medication, food, or fluids

negative reinforcer: any stimulus contingent upon a response, the withdrawal of which results in an increase in the frequency of the response

neuron: the basic nerve cell of the nervous system, containing a nucleus within a cell body. Sensory neurons transmit nerve impulses to the spinal cord and the brain. Motor neurons transmit impulses from the brain to the muscles. All neurons have at least one axon and one or more dendrites.

neurotransmitters: any one of numerous chemicals that modify or result in the transmission of nerve impulses between synapses. Neurotransmitters are released from synaptic knobs (end feet) into synaptic clefts and bridge the gap between neurons. When a nerve impulse reaches a synaptic knob, thousands of neurotransmitter molecules squirt into the synaptic cleft and bind to specific receptors.

Node of Ranvier: a space separating the Schwann cells that form the covering or myelin on a nerve axon

noninvasive: of or pertaining to a diagnostic or therapeutic technique that does not require the skin to be broken or a cavity or organ to be entered

olfactory: of or pertaining to the sense of smell

operant conditioning: a process in which the frequency of a behavior is modified by the consequence that follows. The principles of reinforcement are the techniques used to modify the relationships between an organism and its environment.

optic chiasm: the point at which the optic nerve from one eye crosses to join the other

pathognomonic signs: a variety of indicators which suggest neuro-psychological dysfunction

peripheral nerves: nerves that lie outside the brain and spinal cord

pons: a prominence on the brain stem located between the medulla oblongata and the midbrain. The pons, which consists of white matter and a few nuclei, plays a part in the coordination of postural and kinesthetic information and helps to regulate motor impulses.

positive reinforcer: any stimulus contingent upon a response, the presentation of which results in an increase in the frequency of that response

positron emission tomography (PET): a computerized radiographic technique that employs radioactive substances to examine the metabolic activity of various body structures. In PET studies, the patient either inhales or is injected a biochemical, such as glucose, that emits positively charged particles that combine with negatively charged electrons normally found in the cells of the body. This combination emits gamma rays which are detected and converted to color-coded images by the PET computers.

posterior: of or pertaining to the back part of a structure

post traumatic amnesia (PTA): the interval between the injury and the point at which a patient begins to lay down continuous memory

pragmatics: communication in context. Encompasses ways in which context is used to convey information and how a speaker manipulates nonverbal and verbal messages to express an intention

prefrontal cortex: the tertiary or association areas of the frontal lobes

premorbid: prior to the onset of illness or injury

prophylactic: an agent that prevents the spread of disease

proprioception: sensation pertaining to stimuli originating from within the body regarding spatial position and muscular activity or to the sensory receptors they activate

prosody: the intonation and stress patterns of a verbal message

punishment: the withdrawal of a positive reinforcer or the presentation of a negative reinforcer which results in a reduction of the targeted response

putamen: a nucleus of the basal ganglia complex

reticular formation: a small thick band of neurons within the brain stem that controls breathing, blood pressure, heart beat, level of consciousness, and other vital functions. The reticular formation constantly monitors the state of the body through its connections with sensory and motor tracts

retrograde amnesia: inability to remember events that occurred prior to the onset of amnesia

retrograde memory: memory for events that preceded the injury

rigidity: a condition of stiffness, hardness, or inflexibility

roentgenograms: photography using X-rays

Schwann cells: glial cells that form myelin in the peripheral nervous system

sequelae: the pathological consequences that follow a traumatic insult or onset of disease

shaping: the gradual modification of a response through the reinforcement of successive approximations toward a desired goal

shearing: refers to the type of brain lesion often seen as a result of an abrupt deceleration in movement which causes a continuation of brain movement within the skull. Shearing lesions are recognized as tears in nerve fibers, particularly of axons through the white matter.

spasticity: a condition of spasms or other uncontrolled contractions of the skeletal muscles

stereognosis: an impaired ability to recognize objects by the sense of touch

stimulation therapy: a form of aphasia therapy that aims to stimulate responses by means of repetition and auditory stimulation. Patients are involved in activities that make use of classes of words, similar sounding words, etc. Everyday situations are practiced to develop and stimulate communication.

synapse: the area surrounding the point of contact between two neurons across which nerve impulses are transmitted through the action of a neurotransmitter. Synapses are polarized so that nerve impulses travel in only one direction. Fatigue, oxygen deficiency, and chemical agents can affect the efficiency of the synapses.

time out: in behavioral terms, a period of nonreinforcement usually arranged by removing the opportunity for reinforcing consequences

tracheostomy: an incision through the neck into the trachea with a tube inserted to establish airway

traumatic head injury (THI): mild to severe adventitious brain injury and associated dysfunction produced by a definite blow or wound to the head

tremor: rhythmic, purposeless, quivering movements resulting from the involuntary alternating contraction and relaxation of opposing groups of muscles

ventilator: machine that aids breathing by moving air in and out of the lungs through the endotracheal or tracheostomy tube

ventricles: the cavities of the brain that contain cerebrospinal fluid

ventriculography: an X-ray examination of the head following the injection of air or another contrast medium into the cerebral ventricles

ventriculostomy: insertion of small tube within one of the fluid-filled ventricles

Visual Communication Therapy: a method used to teach language to globally aphasic patients by means of simple figural and geometric symbols originally used to train chimpanzees

Wernicke's aphasia: an aphasia characterized by severe deficits in auditory comprehension resulting from a lesion to Wernicke's area of the brain

white matter: those areas of the nervous system rich in axons covered with glial cells

REFERENCES

Abreu, B. (1985, March). Perceptual cognitive rehabilitation: An occupational therapy model. *Physical Disabilities: Special Interest Section Newsletter.* The American Occupational Therapy Association, *8*(1), pp. 1, 2, 3.

Achenbach, T. M., & Edelbrock, C. S. (1986). *Child Behavior Checklist and Youth Self-Report.* Burlington, VT: Author.

Adamovich, B. B., Henderson, J. A,. & Auerbach, S. (1985). *Cognitive rehabilitation of closed head injured patients: A dynamic approach.* San Diego: College-Hill Press.

Albert, M. L., Sparks, R. W., & Helm, N. A. (1973). Melodic intonation therapy for aphasia. *Archives of Neurology, 29,* 130-131.

Alderman, N., & Burgess, P. W. (1990). Integrating cognition and behavior: A pragmatic approach to brain injury rehabilitation. In R. L. Wood & I. Fussey (Eds.), *Cognitive rehabilitation in perspective* (pp. 204-228). London: Taylor & Frances.

Alexander, M. P. (1984). Neurobehavioral consequences of closed head injury. *Neurology and Neurosurgery, 5*(20), 1-8.

Alves, W. M., & Jane, J. A. (1985). Mild brain injury: Damage and outcome. In D. Becker & J. T. Povlishock (Eds.), *Central nervous system trauma: Status report* (pp. 255-271). Bethesda, MD: National Institutes of Health, National Institute of Neurological and Communicative Disorders and Stroke.

Ambrose, J., Gooding, M. R., & Uttley, D. (1976). EMI scan in the management of injuries. *Lancet, i,* 847-848.

Anastasi, A. (1982). *Psychological testing* (5th ed.). New York: Macmillan.

Anderson, D. P., & Ford, R. M. (1980). Visual abnormalities after severe head injuries. *Canadian Journal of Surgery, 23,* 163-165.

Avidan, R. (1977). Self-care training for patients with hemiplegia, Parkinsonism, and arthritis. In R. D. Sine, S. E. Liss, R. E. Roush, & J. D. Holcomb (Eds.), *Basic rehabilitation techniques: A self-instructional guide* (pp. 127-160). Germantown, MD: Aspen Systems.

HEAD INJURY IN CHILDREN AND ADOLESCENTS

Axelrod, D. (1986). *Head injury in New York State: A report to Governor Cuomo and the legislature.* Albany, NY: Office of Health Care Systems Management, Division of Health Care Standards and Surveillance.

Ayres, A. J. (1972). *Sensory intégration and learning disorders.* Los Angeles: Western Psychological Services.

Bach-y-Rita, P. (1981). Brain plasticity as a basis for development of rehabilitation procedures for hemiplegia. *Scandinavian Journal of Rehabilitative Medicine, 13,* 73-83.

Bagby, G. (1991, Winter). Advances in anticonvulsant therapy. *Headlines,* 2-5, 7-8.

Bakay, L., & Glasauer, F. E. (1980). *Head injury.* Boston: Little, Brown & Co.

Baker, L. L., Parker, K., & Sanderson, D. (1983). Neuromuscular electrical stimulation for the head injured patient. *Physical Therapy, 63,* 1967-1974.

Barin, J. J., Hanchett, J. M., Jacob, W. L., & Scott, M. B. (1985). Counseling the head injured patient. In M. Ylvisaker (Ed.), *Head injury rehabilitation: Children and adolescents* (pp. 361-383). San Diego: College-Hill Press.

Barth, J. T., & Boll, T. J. (1981). Rehabilitation and treatment of central nervous system dysfunction: A behavioral medicine perspective. In C. Prokop & L. Bradley (Eds.), *Medical psychology: Contributions to behavioral medicine.* New York: Academic Press.

Barth, J. T., & Macciocchi, S. N. (1985). The Halstead-Reitan Neuropsychological Test Battery. In C. Newmark (Ed.), *Major psychological assessment techniques* (pp. 381-414). Boston: Allyn & Bacon.

Baxter, R., Cohen, S., & Ylvisaker, M. (1985). Comprehensive cognitive assessment. In M. Ylvisaker (Ed.), *Head injury rehabilitation: Children and adolescents* (pp. 247-275). San Diego: College-Hill Press.

Beaumont, J. (1983). *Introduction to neuropsychology.* New York: Guilford Press.

Becker, B. (1975). Intellectual changes after closed head injury. *Journal of Clinical Psychology, 31,* 307-309.

Becker, D. P., Miller, J. D., Ward, J. D., Greenberg, R. P., Young, H. F., & Sakalas, R. (1977). The outcome from severe head injury with early diagnosis and intensive management. *Journal of Neurosurgery, 47,* 491-502.

Beery, K. (1967). *Developmental Test of Visual-Motor Integration.* Chicago: Follett Education Corporation.

Begali, V. (1987). *Head injury in children and adolescents: A resource and review for school and allied professionals.* Brandon, VT: Clinical Psychology Publishing.

Begali, V. (in press). The role of assessment following traumatic brain injury. In R. C. Savage & G. F. Wolcott (Eds.), *Educational programming for children and young adults with acquired brain injuries.* San Diego: College-Hill Press.

Bellak, L., & Bellak, S. (1974). *Children's Apperception Test.* San Antonio: The Psychological Corporation.

Bender, L. (1974). *Manual for instruction and test cards for Visual Motor Gestalt Test.* New York: American Orthopsychiatric Association.

References

Bennett, T. (1988). Use of the Halstead-Reitan Neuropsychological Test Battery in the assessment of head injury. *Cognitive Rehabilitation, 6*(3), 18-24.

Benton, A. L. (1965). *Sentence Memory Test.* Iowa City: Author.

Benton, A. L. (1974). *The Revised Visual Retention Test* (4th ed.). New York: Psychological Association.

Benton, A. L. (1978). Visuoperceptive, visuospatial, and visuoconstructive disorders. In K. M. Heilman & E. Valenstein (Eds.), *Clinical neuropsychology.* Oxford: Oxford University Press.

Benton, A. L. (1979a). The neuropsychological significance of finger recognition. In M. Bortner (Ed.), *Cognitive growth and development* (pp. 85-105). New York: Brunner/Mazel.

Benton, A. L. (1979b). Behavioral consequences of closed head injury. *Central Nervous System Status Report* (pp. 220-231). Bethesda, MD: National Institutes of Health, National Institute of Neurological and Communicative Disorders and Stroke.

Benton, A. L., & Hamsher, K. (1978). *Multilingual Aphasia Examination.* Iowa City: University of Iowa.

Benton, A. L., Hamsher, K., Varney, N. R., & Spreen, O. (1983). *Contributions to neuropsychological assessment: A clinical manual.* New York: Oxford University Press.

Benton, A. L., Levin, H. S., & Van Allen, M. W. (1974). Geographic orientation in patients with unilateral cerebral disease. *Neuropsychologia, 12,* 183-191.

Ben-Yishay, Y. (1980). *Working approaches to remediation of cognitive deficits in brain-damaged patients* (Rehabilitation Monograph No. 61). New York: New York University Medical Center, Institute of Rehabilitation Medicine.

Ben-Yishay, Y., & Diller, L. (1983). Cognitive remediation. In M. Rosenthal, E. Griffith, M. Bond, & D. Miller (Eds.), *Rehabilitation of the head-injured adult* (pp. 367-380). Philadelphia: F. A. Davis.

Ben-Yishay, Y., Diller, L., Gerstman, L., & Gordon, W. (1970). Relationship between initial competence and ability to profit from cues in brain-damaged individuals. *Journal of Abnormal Psychology, 75,* 248-259.

Ben-Yishay, Y., & Gold, J. (1990). Therapeutic milieu approach to neuropsychological rehabilitation. In R. L. Wood (Ed.), *Neurobehavioral sequelae of traumatic brain injury* (pp. 194-215). New York: Taylor & Frances.

Ben-Yishay, Y., Rattok, J., Ross, B., Lakin, P., Ezrachi, O., Silver, S., & Diller, L. (1982). Rehabilitation of cognitive and perceptual defects in people with traumatic brain damage: A five-year clinical research study. In *Working approaches to remediation of cognitive deficits in brain-damaged persons* (Rehabilitation Monograph No. 64) (pp. 127-176). New York: New York University Medical Center: Institute of Rehabilitation Medicine.

The best yardstick we have. (1961). *Lancet, ii,* 1445-1446.

Binder, L. M., & Rattok, J. (1989). Assessment of the postconcussive syndrome after mild head trauma. In M. D. Lezak (Ed.), *Assessment of the behavioral consequences of head trauma* (pp. 37-48). New York: Alan R. Liss.

Black, P., Blumer, D., Wellner, A. M., & Walker, A. E. (1971). The head-injured child: Timecourse of recovery. In *Head injuries: Proceedings of an International Symposium.* Edinburgh, Madrid; Baltimore: Williams & Wilkins.

Blazyk, S. (1983). Developmental crisis in adolescents following severe head injury. *Social Work in Health Care, 8*(4), 55-67.

Blosser, J., & DePompei, R. (1989). The head injured student returns to school: Recognizing and treating deficits. *Topics in Language Disorders, 9*(2), 67-77.

Blumer, D., & Benson, D. F. (1975). Personality changes in frontal and temporal lobe lesions. In D. F. Benson & D. Blumer (Eds.), *Psychiatric aspects of neurologic disorders.* New York: Grune & Stratton.

Boder, E. (1973). Developmental dyslexia: A diagnostic approach based on three atypical reading-spelling patterns. *Developmental Medicine and Child Neurology, 15,* 663-687.

Bolger, J. P. (1982). Cognitive retraining: A developmental approach. *Clinical Neuropsychology, 4*(2), 66-70.

Boll, T. J. (1978). Diagnosing brain impairment. In B. B. Wolman (Ed.), *Clinical diagnosis of mental disorders* (pp. 601-675). New York: Plenum Press.

Boll, T. J. (1982). Behavioral sequelae of head injury. In P. Cooper (Ed.), *Head injury* (pp. 363-377). Baltimore: Williams & Wilkins.

Boll, T. J. (1983). Minor head injury in children—out of sight but not out of mind. *Journal of Clinical Psychology, 12,* 74-80.

Boll, T. J., & Barth, J. T. (1981). Neuropsychology of brain damage in children. In S. Filskov & T. J. Boll (Eds.), *Handbook of neuropsychology* (pp. 418-453). New York: Wiley.

Boller, F., & Frank, E. (1981). *Sexual functions in neurological disorders.* New York: Raven Press.

Bolton, B. (1982). *Vocational adjustment of the disabled.* Baltimore: University Park Press.

Bond, M. R. (1975). Psychosocial outcome after severe head injury. *Ciba Foundation Symposium, 34,* 145-153.

Bond, M. (1983). Standardized methods of assessing and predicting outcome. In M. Rosenthal, E. R. Griffith, M. R. Bond, & J. D. Miller (Eds.), *Rehabilitation of the head injured adult* (pp. 97-117). Philadelphia: F. A. Davis.

Bornstein, R. A., & Matarazzo, J. D. (1982). Wechsler VIQ versus PIQ differences in cerebral dysfunction: A literature review with emphasis on sex differences. *Journal of Clinical Neuropsychology, 4,* 319-334.

Bowers, S. A., & Marshall, L. F. (1980). Outcome in 200 consecutive cases of severe head injury treated in San Diego County: A prospective analysis. *Neurosurgery, 6,* 234-242.

Boyd, R. D. (1974). *The Boyd Development Progress Scale.* San Bernardino, CA: Inland Counties Regional Center.

Braakman, R., Gelpke, G. J., Habbema, J. D., Mass, A. I., & Minderhoud, J. M. (1980). Systematic selection of prognostic features in patients with severe head injury. *Neurosurgery, 6*(4), 362-370.

References

Bracy, O. (1983). Computer-based cognitive rehabilitation. *Cognitive Rehabilitation*, *1*(1), 7-8.

Bracy, O. (1985). *Programs for cognitive rehabilitation* (catalog). Indianapolis: Psychological Software Services.

Brink, J. D., Garrett, A. L., Hale, W. R., Woo-Sam, J., & Nickel, V. C. (1970). Recovery of motor and intellectual function in children sustaining severe injuries. *Developmental Medicine Child Neurology*, *12*, 565-571.

Brink, J. D., Imbus, C., & Woo-Sam, J. (1980). Physical recovery after severe closed head trauma in children and adolescents. *Journal of Pediatrics*, *97*, 721-727.

Brinkman, S. D. (1979). Rehabilitation of the neurologically impaired patient: The contribution of the neuropsychologist. *Clinical Neuropsychology*, *1*, 39-44.

Broca, P. (1865). Sur le siège de la faculté du langage articulé. *Bulletin of the Society of Anthropology*, *6*, 377-396.

Brooks, D. N. (1976). Wechsler Memory Scale performance and its relationship to brain damage after severe closed head injury. *Journal of Neurology, Neurosurgery, and Psychiatry*, *39*, 593-601.

Brooks, D. N. (1987). Measuring neuropsychological and functional recovery. In H. S. Levin, J. Grafman, & H. M. Eisenberg (Eds.), *Neurobehavioral recovery from head injury* (pp. 57-72). New York: Oxford University Press.

Brooks, D. N., & Aughton, M. E. (1979). Psychological consequences of blunt head injury. *International Rehabilitative Medicine*, *1*, 160.

Brooks, D. N., & McKinlay, W. (1983). Personality and behavioral change after severe blunt head injury—a relative's view. *Journal of Neurology, Neurosurgery, and Psychiatry*, *46*, 333-334.

Brookshire, R. H. (1978). *An introduction to aphasia* (2nd ed.). Minneapolis, MN: BRK Publishers.

Brown, G., Chadwick, O., Shaffer, D., Rutter, M., & Traub, M. (1981). A prospective study of children with head injuries: III. Psychiatric sequelae. *Psychological Medicine*, *11*, 63-78.

Bruce, D. A. (1983). Clinical care of the severely head-injured child. In K. Shapiro (Ed.), *Pediatric head trauma* (pp. 27-44). New York: Futura.

Bruce, D., Schut, L., Bruno, L. A., Wood, J. H., & Sutton, L. N. (1978). Outcome following severe head injury in children. *Journal of Neurosurgery*, *48*, 679-688.

Brudny, J., Korein, J., Bruce, D. A., Grynbaum, B. B., Belandres, P. V., & Gianutsos, J. (1979). Helping hemiparetics to help themselves: Sensory feedback therapy. *Journal of American Medical Association*, *241*, 814-818.

Buck, M. W. (1968). *Dysphasia*. Englewood Cliffs, NJ: Prentice-Hall.

Buffery, A. W. (1977). Clinical neuropsychology: A review and preview. In S. Rachman (Ed.), *Contribution to medical psychology* (pp. 115-137). Oxford: Pergamon Press.

Burgemeister, B. B., Blum, L. H., & Lorge, I. (1972). *Columbia Mental Maturity Scale*. San Antonio: The Psychological Corporation.

Burgess, P. W., & Wood, R. L. (1990). Neuropsychology of behavior disorders following brain injury. In R. L. Wood (Ed.), *Neurobehavioral sequelae of traumatic brain injury* (pp. 110-133). New York: Taylor & Frances.

Burns, P. G., Cook, J., & Ylvisaker, M. (1988). Cognitive assessment and intervention. In R. C. Savage & G. F. Wolcott (Eds.), *An educator's manual: What educators need to know about students with traumatic brain injury* (pp. 25-51). Southborough, MA: National Head Injury Foundation.

Burns, P., & Gianutsos, R. (1987). Re-entry of the head-injured survivor into the educational system. *Journal of Community Health Nursing, 4*(3), 145-152.

Burton, L. (1968). *Vulnerable children.* New York: Schocken Books.

Buschke, H., & Fuld, P. A. (1974). Evaluating storage, retention, and retrieval in disordered memory and learning. *Neurology, 24,* 1019-1025.

Bush, W. J., & Giles, M. T. (1969). *Aids to psycholinguistic teaching.* Columbus, OH: Charles E. Merrill.

Campbell, S. B. (1976). Hyperactivity: Course and treatment. In A. Davids (Ed.), *Child personality and psychology: Current topics, 3.* New York: Wiley.

Caplan, B. (1982). Neuropsychology and rehabilitation. Its role in evaluation and intervention. *Archives of Physical Medicine and Rehabilitation, 63,* 362-366.

Cardenas, D. D. (1987). Antipsychotics and their use after traumatic brain injury. *Journal of Head Trauma Rehabilitation, 2*(4), 43-49.

Carrow-Woolfolk, E. (1985). *Test for Auditory Comprehension of Language.* Allen, TX: DLM.

Cartlidge, N. E. F., & Shaw, D. A. (1981). *Head injury.* London: W. B. Saunders.

Cassidy, J. W. (1990). Pharmacological treatment of behavioral disorders: Aggression and disorder of mood. In R. L. Wood (Ed.), *Neurobehavioral sequelae of traumatic head injury* (pp. 219-249). New York: Taylor & Frances.

Castelnuovo-Tedesco, P. (1984). Psychological consequences of physical defect and trauma. In D. W. Krueger (Ed.), *Emotional rehabilitation of physical trauma and disability* (pp. 25-35). New York: SP Medical & Scientific Books.

Caveness, W. F. (1979). Incidence of craniocerebral trauma in the US in 1976 with trends from 1970-1975. In R. A. Thompson & J. R. Green (Eds.), *Advances in neurology* (pp. 1-3). New York: Raven Press.

Cereghino, J. J. (1990). Treatment implications from classification of seizures and the epilepsies. In D. B. Smith (Ed.), *Epilepsy: Current approaches to diagnosis and treatment* (pp. 1-25). New York: Raven Press.

Chadwick, O., & Rutter, M. (1983). Neuropsychological assessment. In M. Rutter (Ed.), *Developmental neuropsychiatry* (pp. 181-213). New York: Guilford Press.

Chadwick, O., Rutter, M., & Brown, G. (1981). A prospective study of children with head injuries. *Psychological Medicine, 11,* 49-61.

Chadwick, O., Rutter, M., Shaffer, D., & Shrout, P. E. (1981). A prospective study of children with head injuries: IV. Specific cognitive deficits. *Journal of Clinical Neuropsychology, 3,* 101-120.

References

Chadwick, O., Rutter, M., Thompson, J., & Shaffer, D. (1981). Intellectual performance and reading ability after localized head injury in childhood. *Journal of Child Psychology and Psychiatry, 22*, 117-139.

Chamovitz, I., Chorazy, A. J., Hanchett, J. M., & Mandella, P. (1985). Rehabilitative medical management. In M. Ylvisaker (Ed.), *Head injury rehabilitation: Children and adolescents* (pp. 117-141). San Diego: College-Hill Press.

Chelune, G., Ferguson, W., & Moehle, K. (1986). The role of standard cognitive and personality tests in neuropsychological assessment. In T. Incagnoli, G. Goldstein, & C. Golden (Eds.), *Clinical application of neuropsychological test batteries* (pp. 75-119). New York: Plenum Press.

Christensen, A., & Rosenberg, N. K. (1991). A critique of the role of psychotherapy in brain injury rehabilitation. *Journal of Head Trauma Rehabilitation, 6*(4), 56-61.

Cicerone, K. D. (1991). Psychotherapy after mild traumatic brain injury: Relation to the nature and severity of subjective complaints. *Journal of Head Trauma Rehabilitation, 6*(4), 30-43.

Cicerone, K. D., & Wood, J. C. (1987). Planning disorder after closed injury: A case study. *Archives of Physical Medicine and Rehabilitation, 68*, 111-115.

Cicerone, K. D., & Tupper, D. E. (1986). Cognitive assessment in the neuropsychological rehabilitation of head-injured adults. In B. P. Uzzell & Y. Gross (Eds.), *Clinical neuropsychology of intervention* (pp. 59-83). Boston: Martinus Nijhoff.

Cohen, S., Joyce, C., Rhoades, K., & Welks, D. (1985). Educational programming for head injured students. In M. Ylvisaker (Ed.), *Head injury rehabilitation: Children and adolescents* (pp. 383-411). San Diego: College-Hill Press.

Conners, C. K. (1985). *Conners Rating Scales.* San Antonio: The Psychological Corporation.

Cooper, P. (1982). Post-traumatic intracranial mass lesions. In P. Cooper (Ed.), *Head injury* (pp. 185-233). Baltimore: Williams & Wilkins.

Cope, D. N. (1986). The pharmacology of attention and memory. *Journal of Head Trauma Rehabilitation, 1*(3), 34-42.

Cope, D. N. (1987). Psychopharmacologic consideration in the treatment of brain injury. *Journal of Head Trauma Rehabilitation, 2*(4), 1-5.

Cope, D. N. (1990). Pharmacology for behavioral deficits: Disorders of cognition and affect. In R. L. Wood (Ed.), *Neurobehavioral sequelae of traumatic head injury* (pp. 250-273). New York: Taylor & Frances.

Corkin, S. (1968). Acquisition of motor skill after bilateral medical temporal lobe excision. *Neuropsychologia, 6*, 255-266.

Costello, J. (1977). Programmed instruction. *Journal of Speech Hearing Disorders, 42*, 3-28.

Crovitz, H. F., Harvey, M. T., & Horn, R. W. (1979). Problems in the acquisition of imagery mnemonics: Three brain-damaged cases. *Cortex, 15*, 225-234.

Cruikshank, W. M., Bentzen, F. A., Ratzeburg, F. H., & Tannhauser, M. T. (1961). *A teaching method for brain-injured and hyperactive children: A demonstration-pilot study.* Syracuse, NY: Syracuse University Press.

229

Cummings, J. L. (1985). Hemispheric specialization: A history of current concepts. In M. Burns, A. Halper, & S. Mogil (Eds.), *Clinical management of right hemisphere dysfunction* (pp. 1-6). Rockville, MD: Aspen.

Cusick, B. D., & Sussman, M. D. (1981). *Short leg casts: Their role in management of cerebral palsy.* Unpublished manuscript, University of Virginia Children's Medical Center, Charlottesville.

Das, J. P., Kirby, J. P., & Jarman, R. F. (1979). *Simultaneous and successive cognitive processes.* New York: Academic Press.

Davis, J. (1985). Neuronal rearrangements after brain injury. In D. Becker & J. T. Povlishock (Eds.), *Central nervous system trauma: Status report* (pp. 491-503). Bethesda, MD: National Institutes of Health, National Institute of Neurological and Communicative Disorders and Stroke.

Davis, R., & Cunningham, P. S. (1984). Prognostic factors in severe head injury. *Surgery, Gynecology & Obstetrics, 159,* 597-604.

Davis, R. A., & Davis, L. (1982). Decerebrate rigidity in humans. *Neurosurgery, 10,* 635-642.

DePompei, R., & Zarski, J. J. (1989). Families, head injury, and cognitive-communicative impairments: Issues for family counseling. *Topics in Language Disorders, 9*(2), 78-89.

Deelman, B. G., Berg, I., & Koning-Haanstra, M. (1990). Memory strategies for closed head injured patients: Do lessons in cognitive psychology help? In R. L. Wood & I. Fussey (Eds.), *Cognitive rehabilitation in perspective* (pp. 117-144). London: Taylor & Frances.

Dikmen, S., Reitan, R. M., & Temkin, N. R. (1983). Neuropsychological recovery in head injury. *Archives of Neurology, 40,* 333-338.

Diller, L. (1976). A model for cognitive retraining in rehabilitation. *The Clinical Psychologist, 29,* 13-15.

Diller, L. (1980). The development of a perceptual remediation program in hemiplegia. In L. P. Ince (Ed.), *Behavioral psychology in rehabilitation medicine: Clinical applications* (pp. 64-68). Baltimore: Williams & Wilkins.

Diller, L. (1985, March). Results of cognitive rehabilitation. *Physical Disabilities: Special Interest Section Newsletter.* The American Occupational Therapy Association, *8*(1), pp. 1, 4, 5.

Diller, L., & Gordon, W. (1981). Interventions for cognitive deficits in brain-injured adults. *Journal of Consulting and Clinical Psychology, 49,* 822-834.

DiSimoni, F. (1978). *The Token Test for Children.* Boston: Teaching Resources.

Divack, J. A., Herrle, J., & Scott, M. B. (1985). Behavioral management. In M. Ylvisaker (Ed.), *Head injury rehabilitation: Children and adolescents* (pp. 347-360). San Diego: College-Hill Press.

Doronzo, J. F. (1990). Mild head injury. In E. Lehr (Ed.), *Psychological management of traumatic brain injuries in children and adolescents* (pp. 207-224). Rockville, MD: Aspen.

Dunn, L. M. (1981). *Manual for the Peabody Picture Vocabulary Test-Revised.* Circle Pines, MN: American Guidance Service.

References

Dunn, L. M., & Markwardt, F. C. (1970). *Manual for the Peabody Individual Achievement Test*. Circle Pines, MN: American Guidance Service.

Eames, P. (1980, March). *Applications of behavior modification to brain injury*. Paper presented to Third Annual Conference "Head Trauma Rehabilitation Coma to Community," San Jose, CA.

Eames, P. (1990). Organic basis of behavior disorder after traumatic brain injury. In R. L. Wood (Ed.), *Neurobehavioral sequelae of traumatic head injury* (pp. 134-150). New York: Taylor & Frances.

Eisenberg, H. (1985). Outcome after head injury: General considerations and neurobehavioral recovery. In D. Becker & J. T. Povlishock (Eds.), *Central nervous system trauma: Status report* (pp. 271-281). Bethesda, MD: National Institutes of Health, National Institute of Neurological and Communicative Disorders and Stroke.

Elliot, C. C. (1990). *Differential Ability Scales*. San Antonio: The Psychological Corporation.

Elliott, C., Murray, D. J., & Pearson, L. S. (1983). *The British Ability Scales*. San Antonio: The Psychological Corporation.

Ellis, A. (1962). *Reason and emotion in psychotherapy*. New York: Lyle Stuart.

Ellis, A. (1975). *A new guide to rational living*. Hollywood, CA: Wilshire Books.

Engum, E. S., & Lambert, E. W. (1990). Restandardization of the Cognitive Behavioral Driver's Inventory. *Cognitive Rehabilitation, 8*(6), 20-27.

Eson, M. E., & Bourke, R. S. (1980, February). *Assessment of information processing deficits after serious head injury*. Paper presented at the eighth annual meeting of the International Neuropsychological Society, San Francisco, CA.

Evans, R. W., & Gualtieri, C. T. (1987). Psychostimulant pharmacology in traumatic brain injury. *Journal of Head Trauma Rehabilitation, 2*(4), 29-33.

Evans, C. D. (Ed.). (1981). *Rehabilitation after severe head injury*. New York: Churchill Livingstone.

Ewing-Cobbs, L., Fletcher, J. M., & Levin, H. (1985). Neuropsychological sequelae following pediatric head injury. In M. Ylvisaker (Ed.), *Head injury rehabilitation: Children and adolescents* (pp. 3-91). San Diego: College-Hill Press.

Ewing-Cobbs, L., Levin, H. S., Fletcher, J. M., McLaughlin, E. J., McNeely, D. G., Ewert, J., & Francis, D. (1984, February). *Assessment of posttraumatic amnesia in head-injured children*. Paper presented to the International Neuropsychological Society.

Federal Register. (1977). 42 (250), p. 42478.

Federal Register. (1991). 56 (160), p. 41266.

Feeney, D. M., Gonzalez, A., & Law, W. A. (1982). Amphetamine, haloperidol, and experience interact to affect rate of recovery after motor cortex injury. *Science, 217*, 855-857.

Fenichel, G. M. (1988). *Clinical pediatric neurology*. Philadelphia: Saunders.

Fernald, G. (1943). *Remedial techniques in basic school subjects*. New York: McGraw-Hill.

Ferry, P. C., & Cooper, J. (1978). Sign language in communication disorders of children. *Journal of Pediatrics, 93,* 547-552.

Fife, D., Faich, G., Hollingshead, W., & Boynton, W. (1986). Incidence and outcome of hospital-treated head injury in Rhode Island. *American Journal of Public Health, 76*(7), 773-778.

Fitzhugh, K. B., Fitzhugh, L. C., & Reitan, R. M. (1962). Wechsler-Bellevue comparison in groups with "chronic" and "current" lateralized and diffuse brain lesions. *Journal of Consulting and Clinical Psychology, 26,* 306-310.

Flach, J., & Malmros, R. (1972). A long-term follow-up study of children with severe head injury. *Scandinavian Journal of Rehabilitative Medicine, 19,* 495-502.

Flor-Henry, P. (1979). On certain aspects of the localization of the cerebral systems regulating and determining emotion. *Biological Psychiatry, 14,* 677-698.

Fordyce, D. J., Roueche, J. R., & Prigatano, G. P. (1983). Enhanced emotional reaction in chronic head trauma patients. *Journal of Neurology, Neurosurgery, and Psychiatry, 46,* 620-624.

Frankowski, R. F. (1986). Descriptive epidemiologic studies of head injury in the United States: 1974-1984. *Advances in Psychosomatic Medicine, 16,* 153-172.

Frankowski, R. F., Annegers, J. F., & Whitman, S. (1985). Epidemiological and descriptive studies: Part I. In D. Becker & J. T. Povlishock (Eds.), *Central nervous system trauma: Status report* (pp. 33-45). Bethesda, MD: National Institutes of Health, National Institute of Neurological and Communicative Disorders and Stroke.

French, J. L. (1964). *Pictorial Test of Intelligence.* New York: Houghton-Mifflin.

Friedman, A. H. (1983). Head injuries: Initial evaluation and management. *Postgraduate Medicine, 70,* 219-222.

Frowein, R. A. (1976). Classification of coma. *Acta Neurochir, 34,* 5-10.

Fuller, G. B. (1982). *Minnesota Percepto-Diagnostic Test.* Brandon, VT: Clinical Psychology Publishing.

Gaidolfi, E., & Vignolo, L. A. (1980). Closed-head injuries of school-aged children: Neuropsychological sequelae in early adulthood. *Italian Journal of Neurological Science, 1,* 65-73.

Gardner, H., Strub, R., & Albert, M. L. (1975). A unimodal deficit in operational thinking. *Brain and Language, 2,* 333-344.

Gardner, H., Zurif, E. B., Berry, T., & Baker. E. (1976). Visual communication in aphasia. *Neuropsychologia, 14,* 275-292.

Gardner, M. F. (1990). *Expressive One-Word Picture Vocabulary Test-Revised.* Novato, CA: Academic Therapy Publications.

Gates, A. I., & MacGinities, W. H. (1969). *Gates-MacGinities Reading Tests.* New York: Teachers College Press, Columbia University.

Gazzangia, M. S. (1970). *The bisected brain.* New York: Appleton.

Gelfand, D. M., & Hartmann, D. P. (1984). *Child behavior analysis and therapy.* New York: Pergamon Press.

References

Gennarelli, T. A. (1982). Cerebral concussion and diffuse brain injuries. In P. Cooper (Ed.), *Head injury* (pp. 83-89). Baltimore: Williams & Wilkins.

German, D. J. (1990). *Test of Adolescent Word Finding*. Allen, TX: DLM.

Geschwind, N. (1974a). Late changes in the nervous system: An overiew. In D. G. Stein, J. J. Rosen, & N. Butters (Eds.), *Plasticity and recovery of function in the central nervous system* (pp. 467-509). New York: Academic Press.

Geschwind, N. (1974b). The anatomical basis of hemispheric differentiation. In S. J. Diamond & J. C. Beaumont (Eds.), *Hemispheric function in the human brain*. New York: Wiley.

Geschwind, N., & Fusillo, M. (1966). Color naming defects in association with alexia. *Archives of Neurology, 15,* 137-146.

Gheorghita, N. (1981). Vertical reading: A new method of therapy for reading disturbances in aphasics. *Journal of Clinical Neuropsychology, 3,* 161-164.

Gianutsos, R. (1988). *Driving Advisement System*. Bayport, NY: Life Science Associates.

Glasgow, R. E., Zeiss, R. A., Barrera, M., Jr., & Lewinsohn, P. M. (1977). Case studies on remediating memory deficits in brain-damaged individuals. *Journal of Clinical Psychology, 33,* 1049-1054.

Glass, A. V., Gazzangia, M. S., & Premack, D. (1973). Artificial language training in global aphasics. *Neuropsychologia, 11,* 95-103.

Glenn, M. B., & Joseph, A. B. (1987). The use of lithium for behavioral and affective disorders after traumatic brain injury. *Journal of Head Trauma Rehabilitation, 2*(4), 68-76.

Glenn, M. B., & Wroblewski, B. (1989). The choice of antidepressants in depressed survivors of traumatic brain injury. *Journal of Head Trauma Rehabilitation, 4*(3), 85-88.

Godersky, J. C., Gentry, L., Trandel, D., Dyste, G., & Danks, K. (1990). MRI and neurobehavioral outcome in traumatic brain injury. *Acta Neurochirugica Supplement, 51,* 311-314.

Goethe, K., & Levin, H. S. (1984). Behavioral manifestations during early and long-term stages of recovery after closed head injury. *Psychiatric Annals, 14*(7), 540-546.

Goldberger, M. E. (1974). Recovery of movement after CNS lesions in monkeys. In D. G. Stein, J. J. Rosen, & N. Butters (Eds.), *Plasticity and recovery of function in the central nervous system* (pp. 265-339). New York: Academic Press.

Golden, C. J. (1979). *Clinical interpretation of objective psychological tests*. New York: Grune & Stratton.

Golden, C. J. (1981a). *Diagnosis and rehabilitation in clinical neuropsychology*. Springfield, IL: Charles C. Thomas.

Golden, C. J. (1981b). The Luria-Nebraska Children's Battery: Theory and formulation. In G. Hynd & J. Obrzut (Eds.), *Neuropsychological assessment and the school-aged child: Issues and procedures* (pp. 227-302). New York: Grune & Stratton.

Golden, C. (1987). *Luria-Nebraska Neuropsychological Battery: Children's Revision*. Los Angeles: Western Psychological Services.

Golden, C. (1988). Using the Luria-Nebraska neuropsychological examination in cognitive rehabilitation. *Cognitive Rehabilitation, 6*(3), 26-30.

Golden, C., Hammeke, T. A., & Purisch, A. (1980). *Manual for the Luria-Nebraska Neuropsychological Battery*. Los Angeles: Western Psychological Corporation.

Golden, C., & Maruish, M. (1986). The Luria-Nebraska neuropsychological battery. In T. Incagnoli, G. Goldstein, & C. Golden (Eds.), *Clinical application of neuropsychological test batteries* (pp. 193-233). New York: Plenum Press.

Golden, C. J., Moses, J. A. Coffman, J., Miller, W. R., & Strider, F. D. (1983). *Clinical neuropsychology*. New York: Grune & Stratton.

Golden, C., Purisch, A., & Hammeke, T. A. (1985). *Manual for the Luria-Nebraska Neuropsychological Battery–Form II*. Los Angeles: Western Psychological Corporation.

Goldman, P. S. (1974a). An alternative to developmental plasticity: Neurology of CNS structure in infants and adults. In D. G. Stein, J. J. Rosen, & N. Butters (Eds.), *Plasticity and recovery of function in the central nervous system* (pp. 149-175). New York: Academic Press.

Goldman, P. S. (1974b). Recovery of function after CNS lesions in infant monkeys. *Neurosciences Research Program Bulletin, 12*, 217-222.

Goldstein, A. P., Sprafkin, R. P., Gershaw, N. J., & Klein, P. (1980). *Skillstreaming the adolescent: A structured learning approach to teaching social skills*. Champaign, IL: Research Press.

Goldstein, F. C., & Levin, H. S. (1985). Intellectual and academic outcome following closed head injury in children and adolescents: Research strategies and empirical findings. *Developmental Neuropsychology, 1*(3), 195-214.

Goldstein, G. (1984). Neuropsychological assessment. In G. Goldstein & M. Hersen (Eds.), *Handbook of psychological assessment* (pp. 181-211). New York: Pergamon Press.

Goldstein, G. (1986). An overview of the similarities and differences between the Halstead-Reitan and Luria-Nebraska neuropsychological batteries. In T. Incagnoli, G. Goldstein, & C. Golden (Eds.), *Clinical application of neuropsychological test batteries* (pp. 235-275). New York: Plenum Press.

Goldstein, G., & Ruthven, L. (1983). *Rehabilitation of the brain-damaged adult*. New York: Plenum Press.

Goodglass, H., & Kaplan, E. (1972). *The assessment of aphasia and related disorders*. Philadephia: Lea & Febriger.

Goodglass, H., & Kaplan, E. (1979). Assessment of cognitive deficit in the brain-injured patient. In M. S. Gazzangia (Ed.), *Handbook of behavioral neuropsychology (Vol. 2). Neurology* (pp. 1-22). New York: Plenum Press.

Gordon, W. A., Hibbard, M., & Egelko, S. et al. (1985). Perceptual remediation in patients with right brain damage: A comprehensive program. *Archives of Physical and Medical Rehabilitation, 66*, 353-359.

References

Gordon, W. A., Hibbard, M. R., & Kreutzer, J. A. (1989). Cognitive remediation: Issues in research and practice. *Head Trauma Rehabilitation, 4*(3), 76-84.

Grant, D. A., & Berg, E. A. (1980). *Wisconsin Card Sorting Test.* San Antonio: The Psychological Corporation.

Greenberg, R. P., Newlon, P. G., & Hyatt, M. S. (1981). Prognostic implications of early multimodality evoked potentials in severely head-injured patients; a prospective study. *Journal of Neurosurgery, 55,* 227-236.

Gresham, F. M. (1981). Social skills training with handicapped children: A review. *Review of Educational Research, 51,* 139-176.

Griffiths, M. W. (1979). The incidence of auditory and vestibular concussion following minor head injury. *Journal of Laryngology Otology, 93,* 253-265.

Groher, M. (1977). Language and memory disorders following closed head injury. *Journal of Speech and Hearing Research, 20,* 212.

Gronwall, D. M., & Sampson, H. (1974). *The psychological effects of concussion.* Auckland, New Zealand: Auckland University Press.

Gronwall, D., & Wrightson, P. (1974). Delayed recovery of intellectual function after minor head injury. *Lancet, ii,* 605-609.

Gronwall, D., & Wrightson, P. (1975). Cumulative effects of concussion. *Lancet, ii,* 995-997.

Grove, D. N. (1970). *Application of behavioral technology to physical therapy.* Paper presented at the Annual Convention of the American Psychological Association, Miami Beach, FL.

Gualtieri, C. T. (1991). Buspirone: Neuropsychiatric effects. *Journal of Head Trauma Rehabilitation, 6*(1), 90-92.

Gummow, L., Miller, P., & Dustman, R. E. (1983). Attention and brain injury: A case for cognitive rehabilitation of attentional deficits. *Clinical Psychology Review, 3,* 255-274.

Haarbauer-Krupa, J., Henry, K., Szekeres, S., & Ylvisaker, M. (1985). Cognitive rehabilitation therapy: Late stages of recovery. In M. Ylvisaker (Ed.), *Head injury rehabilitation: Children and adolescents* (pp. 311-347). San Diego: College-Hill Press.

Haarbauer-Krupa, J., Moser, L., Smith, C. J., Sullivan, D. M., & Szekeres, S. F. (1985). Cognitive rehabilitation therapy: Middle stages of recovery. In M. Ylvisaker (Ed.), *Head injury rehabilitation: Children and adolescents* (pp. 287-311). San Diego: College-Hill Press.

Haas, J. F. (1987). Ethical and legal aspects of psychotropic medications of brain injury. *Journal of Head Trauma Rehabilitation, 2*(4), 6-17.

Haffey, N. J. (1983). *A demonstration of Luria's qualitative neuropsychological method of cognitive remediation.* Paper presented at the Annual Meeting of the International Neuropsychological Society, Mexico.

Hagen, C. (1981). Language disorders secondary to closed head injury: Diagnosis and treatment. *Topics in Language Disorders, 1,* 73-87.

Hagen, C., Malkmus, D., & Durham, P. (1981). *Rancho Los Amigos: Levels of Cognitive Functioning.* Downey, CA: Professional Staff Association.

Hallahan, D. P., Hall, R., Ianna, S., Kneedler, R., Lloyd, J., Loper, A., & Reeve, R. (1983). Summary of findings at the University of Virginia Learning Disabilities Research Institute. *Exceptional Children Quarterly, 4,* 95-114.

Haller, K., Miller-Meeks, M., & Kardon, R. (1990). Early magnetic resonance imaging in acute traumatic internuclear ophthalmoplegia. *Ophthalmology, 97*(9), 1162-1165.

Halstead, W. C. (1947). *Brain and intelligence.* Chicago: University of Chicago Press.

Halstead, W. C., & Wepman, J. M. (1959). The Halstead-Wepman Aphasia Screening Test. *Journal of Speech and Hearing Disorders, 14,* 9-15.

Hammill, D. D., & Larsen, S. C. (1988). *Test of Written Language.* Chicago: Riverside.

Hanley, I. G. (1982). *A manual for the modification of confused behavior.* Edinburgh: Lothian Regional Council.

Hannay, H. J., Levin, H. S., & Grossman, R. G. (1979). Impaired recognition memory after head injury. *Cortex, 15,* 269-283.

Harley, J. P., Leuthold, C. A., Matthews, C., & Bergs, L. (1980). *Wisconsin Neuropsychological Test Battery.* Madison, WI: C. G. Matthews.

Harris, A. J. (1947). *Harris Tests of Lateral Dominance.* New York: Psychological Corporation.

Hartlage, L. C., & Reynolds, C. R. (1981). Neuropsychological assessment and the individualization of instruction. In G. W. Hynd & J. E. Obrzut (Eds.), *Neuropsychological assessment and the school-aged child: Issues and procedures* (pp. 355-379). New York: Grune & Stratton.

Hauser, W. A., & Hesdorffer, D. C. (1990). *Epilepsy: Frequency, causes and consequences.* Landover, MD: Epilepsy Foundation of America.

Head, H. (1926). *Aphasia and kindred disorders of speech.* New York: Macmillan.

Heaton, R. K., Grant, I., Anthony, W. Z., & Lehman, R. A. W. (1981). A comparison of clinical and automated interpretation of the Halstead-Reitan Battery. *Journal of Clinical Neuropsychology, 3,* 121-141.

Heaton, R. K., & Pendleton, M. G. (1981). Use of neuropsychological tests to predict adult patients' everyday functioning. *Journal of Consulting and Clinical Psychology, 49,* 807-821.

Hebb, D. O. (1942). The effect of early and late brain injury upon test scores, and the nature of normal intelligence. *Proceedings of the American Philosophical Society, 85,* 275.

Hécaen, H. (1976). Acquired aphasia in children and the ontogenesis of hemispheric functional specialization. *Brain Language, 3,* 114-134.

Heilveil, I. (1983). *Video in mental health practice: An activities handbook.* New York: Springer.

Heiskanen, O., & Kaste, M. (1974). Late prognosis of severe brain injury in children. *Developmental Medicine and Child Neurology, 16,* 11-14.

Helffenstein, D. A. (1981). *The effects of interpersonal process recall (IPR) on the interpersonal and communication skills of the newly brain injured.* Unpublished doctoral dissertation, University of Virginia, Charlottesville.

References

Helffenstein, D., & Wechsler, F. (1982). The use of interpersonal process recall (IPR) in the remediation of interpersonal and communication skill deficits in the newly brain-injured. *Clinical Neuropsychology, 4,* 139-143.

Hesse, G. W., & Friedlander, B. Z. (1974). *Behavioral training of a retarded adolescent to develop voluntary use of a previously unused CP involved arm and hand* Unpublished manuscript.

Heward, W. L., & Orlansky, M. D. (1980). *Exceptional children.* Columbus, OH: Charles E. Merrill.

Higashi, K., Sakata, Y., Hatano, M., Abiko, S., Ihara, K., Katayama, S., Wakuta, Y., Okamura, T., Ueda, H., Zenke, M., & Aoki, H. (1977). Epidemiological studies on patients with a persistent vegetative state. *Journal of Neurology, Neurosurgery, and Psychiatry, 40,* 876-885.

Holden, V. P., & Woods, R. T. (1982). *Reality orientation: Psychological approaches to the confused elderly.* London: Churchill Livingstone.

Holland, A. L. (1980). *Communicative Abilities in Daily Living: A test of functional communication for aphasic adults.* Baltimore: University Park Press.

Hollon, T. H. (1973). Behavior modification in a community rehabilitation unit. *Archives of Physical Medicine Rehabilitation, 54,* 65.

Hooper, A. E. (1983). *The Hooper Visual Organization Test Manual.* Los Angeles: Western Psychological Services.

Hopewell, C. A., Burke, W. H., Weslowski, M., & Zawlocki, R. (1990). Behavioral learning therapies for the traumatically brain-injured patient. In R. L. Wood & I. Fussey (Eds.), *Cognitive rehabilitation in perspective* (pp. 229-246). London: Taylor & Frances.

Horn, L. J. (1987). Atypical medications for the treatment of disruptive, aggressive behavior in the brain-injured patient. *Journal of Head Trauma Rehabilitation, 2*(4), 18-28.

Hynd, G. W., & Obrzut, J. E. (Eds.). (1981). *Neuropsychological assessment and the school-aged child: Issues and procedures.* New York: Grune & Stratton.

Incagnoli, T., Goldstein, G., & Golden, C. J. (Eds.). (1986). *Clinical application of neuropsychological test batteries.* New York: Plenum Press.

Ince, L. P. (1969). A behavioral approach to motivation in rehabilitation. *Psychological Records, 19* (105).

Ince, L. P. (1976). *Behavior modification in rehabilitation medicine.* Springfield, IL: Charles C. Thomas.

Ince, L. P., & Rosenberg, D. N. (1973). Modification of articulation in dysarthria. *Archives of Physical and Medical Rehabilitation, 54,* 233.

International Classification of Diseases, Clinical Modification: ICD-9 (9th ed.). (1986). Ann Arbor: Edwards Brothers.

Jaffe, M., Mastrilli, J., Molitor, C. B., & Valko, A. (1985). Physical rehabilitation. In M. Ylvisaker (Ed.), *Head injury rehabilitation: Children and adolescents* (pp. 167-195). San Diego: College-Hill Press.

Jagger, J., Levine, J. I., Jane, J. A., & Rimel, R. W. (1984). Epidemiologic features of head injury in a predominantly rural population. *Journal of Trauma, 24*(1), 40-44.

Jane, J. A., & Rimel, R. W. (1982). Prognosis in head injury. *Clinical Neurosurgery, 29,* 346-352.

Jarvis, P. E., & Barth, J. T. (1984). *Halstead-Reitan Test Battery: An interpretive guide.* Odessa, FL: Psychological Assessment Resources.

Jastak, S., & Wilkinson, G. (1984). *Wide Range Achievement Test-Revised.* Odessa, FL: Psychological Assessment Resources.

Jellinger, K. (1983). The neuropathology of pediatric head injuries. In K. Shapiro (Ed.), *Pediatric head trauma* (pp. 143-194). New York: Futura.

Jennett, B. (1972). Head injuries in childhood. *Developmental Medicine and Child Neurology, 14,* 137.

Jennett, B. (1975a). *Epilepsy after non-missile head injuries.* London: Heinemann Medical Books.

Jennett, B. (1975b). Scale, scope and philosophy of the clinical problem. *Ciba Foundation Symposium, 34,* 3-21.

Jennett, B. (1977). Late effects of head injuries. *Scientific Foundations of Neurology, X,* 441-451.

Jennett, B. (1979). Severity of brain damage: Altered consciousness and other indicators. In G. L. Odom (Ed.), *Central nervous system trauma research status report* (pp. 204-219). Bethesda, MD: National Institutes of Health, National Institute of Neurological and Communicative Disorders and Stroke.

Jennett, B. (1983a). Post traumatic epilepsy. In M. Rosenthal, E. Griffith, M. Bond, & D. Miller (Eds.), *Rehabilitation of the head injured adult* (pp. 119-124). Philadelphia: F. A. Davis.

Jennett, B. (1983b). Scale and scope of the problem. In M. Rosenthal, E. Griffith, M. Bond, & D. Miller (Eds.), *Rehabilitation of the head injured adult* (pp. 3-9). Philadelphia: F. A. Davis.

Jennett, B., & Bond, M. (1975). Assessment of outcome after severe brain damage. *Lancet, i,* 480-487.

Jennett, B., & Teasdale, G. (1981). Management of head injuries. *Contemporary Neurology Series, 20,* 258-260.

Jennett, B., Teasdale, G., Braakman, R., Minderhoud, J., Heiden, J., & Kurze, T. (1979). Prognosis of patients with severe head injury. *Neurosurgery, 4,* 283-289.

Jennett, B., Teasdale, G., Braakman, R., Minderhoud, J., & Knill-Jones, R. (1976). Predicting outcome in individual patients after severe head injury. *Lancet, ii,* 1031-1034.

Johnson, D. J., & Myklebust, H. R. (1967). *Learning disabilities: Educational principles and practices.* New York: Grune & Stratton.

Johnson, G. O., & Boyd, H. F. (1981). *Nonverbal Test of Cognitive Skills.* San Antonio: The Psychological Corporation.

Jones, R., Giddens, H., & Croft, D. (1983). Assessment and training of brain-damaged drivers. *American Journal of Occupational Therapy, 37,* 754-760.

References

Joshi, P., Capozzoli, J. A., & Coyle, J. T. (1985). Effective management with lithium of a persistent, post-traumatic hypomania in a 10-year-old child. *Journal of Developmental and Behavioral Pediatrics, 6*(6), 352-354.

Kagan, N. (1969). Interpersonal process recall. *Journal of Nervous and Mental Disease, 148,* 365-374.

Kagan, N. (1975). *Interpersonal process recall: A method of influencing human interaction.* Mason, MI: Mason Media.

Kagan, N., & Krathwohl, D. R. (1967). *Studies in human interaction: Interpersonal process recall stimulated by videotape.* East Lansing: Educational Publications Services, Michigan State University.

Kahn, R. L., Zarit, S. H., Hilbert, N. M., & Niederehe, G. (1975). Memory complaint and impairment of the aged: The effects of depression and altered brain functions. *Archives of General Psychiatry, 7,* 479-483.

Kalsbeek, W. D., McLaurin, R. L., Harris, B. S., & Miller, J. D. (1980). The national head and spinal cord injury survey: Major findings. In D. W. Anderson & R. L. McLaurin (Eds.), *Report on the national head and spinal cord injury survey* (Contract No. N01-NS-4-2334 and 263-78-C-0132) (pp. 19-31). Bethesda, MD: National Institutes of Health.

Kampen, D. L., & Grafmen, J. (1989). Neuropsychological evaluation of penetrating head injury. In M. D. Lezak (Ed.), *Assessment of the behavioral consequences of head trauma* (pp. 49-60). New York: Alan R. Liss.

Kaplan, E. (1988). A process approach to neuropsychological assessment. In T. Boll & B. K. Bryant (Eds.), *Clinical neuropsychology and brain function* (pp. 125-167). Washington, DC: American Psychological Association.

Kaplan, E., Fein, D., Morris, R., & Delis, D. C. (1991). *Wechsler Adult Intelligence Scale - Revised as a Neuropsychological Instrument.* San Antonio, TX: The Psychological Corporation.

Katz, M. M., & Lyerly, S. B. (1963). Methods of measuring adjustment and social behavior in the community: Rationale, description, discrimination validity, and scale development. *Psychological Reports, 13,* 503.

Kaufman, A. S., & Kaufman, N. (1983). *The Kaufman Assessment Battery for Children.* Circle Pines, MN: American Guidance Service.

Kaufman, A. S., & Kaufman, N. (1985). *Kaufman Test of Educational Achievement.* Circle Pines, MN: American Guidance Service.

Kaufman, H. H., Levin, H. S., High, W. M., Childs, T. L., Wagner, K. A., & Gildenberg, P. L. (1985). Neurobehavioral outcome after gunshot wounds to the head in adult civilians and children. *Neurosurgery, 16,* 754-758.

Kazdin, A. E. (1984). *Behavior modification in applied settings.* Homewood, IL: Dorsey.

Kennedy, R., Bittner, A., & Jones, M. (1981). Video game and conventional tracking. *Perceptual Motor Skills, 93,* 143-152.

Kerr, T. A., Kay, D. W. K., & Lassman, L. P. (1971). Characteristics of patients, type of accident, and mortality in a consecutive series of head injuries admitted to a neurosurgical unit. *British Journal of Preventative Social Medicine, 25,* 179-185.

Kimura, S. D. (1981). A card form of the Reitan-Modified Halstead Category Test. *Journal of Consulting and Clinical Psychology, 49,* 145-146.

Kinsbourne, M., & Hiscock, M. (1981). Cerebral lateralization and cognitive development: Conceptual and methodological issues. In W. Hynd & J. E. Obrzut (Eds.), *Neuropsychological assessment and the school-aged child: Issues and procedures* (pp. 25-167). New York: Grune & Stratton.

Klonoff, H. (1971). Head injuries in children: Predisposing factors, accident conditions, accident proneness, and sequelae. *American Journal of Public Health, 61,* 2405-2417.

Klonoff, H., & Low, M. (1974). Disordered brain function in young children and early adolescents: Neuropsychological and electroencephalographic correlates. In R. M. Reitan & L. A. Davison (Eds.), *Clinical neuropsychology: Current status and applications* (pp. 121-178). New York: Wiley.

Klonoff, H., Low, M. W., & Clark, C. (1977). Head injuries in children: A prospective five year follow-up. *Journal of Neurology, Neurosurgery, and Psychiatry, 40,* 1211-1219.

Klonoff, P., & Prigatano, G. (1987). Reactions of family members and clinical interventions after traumatic brain injury. In M. Ylvisaker & E. M. Gobble (Eds.), *Community re-entry for head-injured adults* (pp. 381-407). Boston: College-Hill Press.

Kohen-Raz, R. (1977). *Psychological aspects of cognitive growth.* New York: Academic Publishing.

Kolb, B., & Whishaw, I. Q. (1980). *Fundamentals of human neuropsychology.* San Francisco: Freeman.

Kolb, B., & Whishaw, I. Q. (1989). *Fundamentals of human neuropsychology - Third edition.* San Francisco: Freeman.

Koppitz, E. M. (1977). *The Visual Aural Digit Span Test.* New York: Grune & Stratton.

Kraus, J. F. (1980). Injury to the head and spinal cord: The epidemiological relevance of the medical literature published from 1960 to 1978. In D. W. Anderson & R. L. McLaurin (Eds.), *Report on the national head and spinal cord injury survey* (Contract No. N01-NS-4-2334 and 263-78-C-0132) (pp. 3-17). Bethesda, MD: National Institutes of Health.

Kraus, J. F. (1989). Epidemiology of head injury. In P. R. Cooper (Ed.), *Head injury* (pp. 1-19). Baltimore: Williams & Wilkins.

Kraus, J. F., Black, M. A., Hessol, N., Ley, P., Rokaw, W., & Sullivan, C. (1984). The incidence of acute brain injury and serious impairments in a defined population. *American Journal of Epidemiology, 119*(2), 186-201.

Krueger, D. W. (1984). Emotional rehabilitation. In D. W. Krueger (Ed.), *Emotional rehabilitation of physical trauma and disability* (pp. 3-12). New York: SP Medical & Scientific Books.

Kubler-Ross, E. (1969). *On death and dying.* New York: Macmillan.

Kurlycheck, R. T., & Glang, A. E. (1984). The use of microcomputers in the cognitive rehabilitation of brain-injured persons. In M. D. Schwartz (Ed.), *Using computers in clinical practice* (pp. 245-256). New York: Haworth Press.

References

Kushner, H., & Knox, A. W. (1973). Application of the utilization technique to the behavior of a brain-injured patient. *Journal of Communication Disorders, 6,* 151.

Lambert, N., Windmiller, M., Tharinger, D., & Cole, L. (1981). *AAMD Adaptive Behavior Scale: School Edition.* Monterey, CA: Publishers Test Service.

Landis, T., Graves, R., Benson D. F., & Hebben, N. (1982). Visual recognition through kinaesthetic mediation. *Psychological Medicine, 12,* 515-531.

Langer, E. J., Rodin, J., Beck, P., Weinman, C., & Spitzer, L. (1979). Environmental determinants of memory improvement in late childhood. *Journal of Personality and Social Psychology, 37*(11), 2003-2013.

Langfitt, T. W., & Gennarelli, T. A. (1982). Can the otucome from head injury be improved? *Journal of Neurosurgery, 56,* 19-25.

Lashley, K. S. (1937). Functional determinants of cerebral localization. *Archives of Neurology and Psychiatry, 38,* 371.

LaVigna, G. W., & Donnellan, A. M. (1986). *Alternatives to punishment: Solving behavior problems with nonaversive strategies.* New York: Irvington.

Lehr, E. (1990a). A developmental perspective. In E. Lehr (Ed.), *Psychological management of traumatic brain injuries in children and adolescents* (pp. 41-98). Rockville, MD: Aspen.

Lehr, E. (1990b). Cognitive aspects. In E. Lehr (Ed.), *Psychological management of traumatic brain injuries in children and adolescents* (pp. 99-132). Rockville, MD: Aspen.

Lehr, E. (1990c). Measurement and process of recovery. In E. Lehr (Ed.), *Psychological management of traumatic brain injuries in children and adolescents* (pp. 15-39). Rockville, MD: Aspen.

Lehr, E. (1990d). Psychosocial issues. In E. Lehr (Ed.), *Psychological management of traumatic brain injuries in children and adolescents* (pp. 155-185). Rockville, MD: Aspen.

Leiter, R. G. (1969). *General instructions for the Leiter International Performance Scale.* Chicago: Stoelting.

Leli, D. A., & Filskov, S. B. (1979). Relationship of intelligence to education and occupation as signs of intellectual deterioration. *Journal of Consulting and Clinical Psychology, 47,* 702-707.

Lenneberg, E. (1967). *Biological foundations of language.* New York: John Wiley.

Levati, A., Farina, M. D., & Vecchi, G. (1982). Prognosis of severe head injuries. *Journal of Neurosurgery, 57,* 779-783.

Levin, H. S. (1978). Behavioral sequelae of closed head injury. *Archives of Neurology, 55,* 720-727.

Levin, H. S. (1985). Outcome after head injury: Part II. In D. Becker & J. T. Povlishock (Eds.), *Central nervous system trauma: Status report* (pp. 281-303). Bethesda, MD: National Institutes of Health, National Institute of Neurological and Communicative Disorders and Stroke.

Levin, H. S. (1990). Predicting the neurobehavioral sequelae of closed head injury. In R. L. Wood (Ed.), *Neurobehavioral sequelae of traumatic brain injury* (pp. 89-109). New York: Taylor & Frances.

HEAD INJURY IN CHILDREN AND ADOLESCENTS

Levin, H. S., Benton, A. L., & Grossman, R. G. (1982). *Neurobehavioral consequences of closed head injury.* New York: Oxford University Press.

Levin, H. S., & Eisenberg, H. M. (1979). Neuropsychological outcome of closed head injury in children and adolescents. In A. J. Raimondi (Ed.), *Child's brain* (pp. 281-292). Basel, Switzerland: S. Karger.

Levin, H. S., Eisenberg, H. M., & Miner, M. E. (1983). Neurophysiologic findings in head injured children. In K. Shapiro (Ed.), *Pediatric head trauma* (pp. 223-240). New York: Futura.

Levin, H. S., Eisenberg, H. M., Wigg, N. R., & Kobayashi, K. (1982). Memory and intellectual ability after head injury in children and adolescents. *Neurosurgery, 11,* 668-673.

Levin, H. S., Ewing-Cobbs, L., & Benton, A. L. (1984). Age and recovery from brain damage. A review of clinical studies. In S. W. Scheff (Ed.), *Aging and recovery of function in the central nervous system* (pp. 169-203). New York: Plenum.

Levin, H. S., & Goldstein, F. C. (1989). Neurobehavioral aspects of traumatic head injury. In P. Bach-y-Rita (Ed.), *Comprehensive neurologic rehabilitation: Vol. 2; Traumatic brain injury* (pp. 53-72). New York: Demos.

Levin, H. S., & Grossman, R. G. (1978). Behavioral sequelae of closed head injury *Archives of Neurology, 35,* 720-727.

Levin, H. S., Grossman, R. G., James, M. D., Rose, M. D., & Teasdale, G. (1979). Long-term neuropsychological outcome of closed head injury. *Journal of Neurosurgery, 50,* 412-422.

Levin, H. S., Grossman, R. G., & Kelly, P. J. (1976). Short-term recognition in memory in relation to severity of head injury. *Cortex, 12,* 175-182.

Levin, H. S., Grossman, R. G., & Kelly, P. J. (1977). Impairment of facial recognition after closed head injuries of varying severity. *Cortex, 13,* 119-130.

Levin, H. S., Grossman, R. G., Rose, J. E., & Teasdale, G. (1979). Long-term neuropsychological outcome of closed head injury. *Journal of Neurosurgery, 50,* 412-422.

Levin, H. S., Grossman, R. G., Sarwar, M., & Meyers, C. A. (1981). Linguistic recovery after closed head injury. *Brain & Language, 12,* 360-374.

Levin, H. S., Kalisky, Z., Handel, S., Goldman, A., Eisenberg, H., Morrison, D., & Von Laufen, A. (1985). Magnetic resonance imaging in relation to the sequelae and rehabilitation of diffuse closed head injury. Preliminary findings. *Seminars in Neurology, 5*(3), 221-231.

Levin, H. S., Meyers, C. A., Grossman, R. G., & Sarwar, M. (1981). Ventricular enlargement of closed head injury. *Archives of Neurology, 38,* 623-629.

Levin, H. S., O'Donnell, V. M., & Grossman, R. G. (1979). The Galveston Orientation and Amnesia Test. A practical scale to assess cognition after head injury. *Journal of Nervous and Mental Diseases, 167,* 675-684.

Levin, H. S., Williams, D., Valastro, M., Eisenberg, H., Crawford, M., & Handel, S. (1990). Corpus callosal atrophy following closed head injury: Detection with MRI. *Journal of Neurosurgery, 73*(1), 77-81.

References

Lewinsohn, P. M., Danaher, B. G., & Kikel, S. (1977). Visual imagery as a mnemonic aid for brain-injured persons. *Journal of Consulting and Clinical Psychology, 45,* 717-723.

Lewis, L. (1991). A framework for developing a psychotherapy treatment plan with brain-injured patients. *Journal of Head Trauma Rehabilitation, 6*(4), 22-29.

Lewis, R. G., & Kupke, T. (1977). *The Lafayette Clinic Repeatable Neuropsychological Test Battery.* Publisher unknown.

Lezak, M. D. (1978). Living with the characterologically altered brain injured patient. *Journal of Clinical Psychiatry, 39,* 592-598.

Lezak, M. D. (1980). *Portland Adaptability Inventory.* New York: Oxford University Press.

Lezak, M. D. (1983). *Neuropsychological assessment.* New York: Oxford University Press.

Lezak, M. D. (1987). Making neuropsychological assessment relevant to head injury. In H. S. Levin, J. Grafman, & H. M. Eisenberg (Eds.), *Neurobehavioral recovery from head injury* (pp. 116-128). New York: Oxford University Press.

Lichtman, M. (1972). *REAL: Reading everyday activities in life.* New York: CAL Press.

Liebman, M. (1986). *Neuroanatomy made easy and understandable.* Rockville, MD: Aspen.

Lishman, W. A. (1968). Brain damage in relation to psychiatric disability after head injury. *British Journal of Psychiatry, 114,* 373-410.

Lishman, W. A. (1973). The psychiatric sequelae of head injury: A review. *Psychological Medicine, 3,* 304-318.

Lishman, W. A. (1978). *Organic psychiatry.* London: Blackwell Scientific Publications.

Lovell, F. M. (1987). Behavioral treatments of aggressive sequelae of brain injury. *Psychiatric Annals, 17*(6), 389-396.

Luria, A. R. (1963). *Restoration of function after brain injury.* New York: Macmillan.

Luria, A. R. (1966). *Higher cortical functions in man.* New York: Basic Books.

Luria, A. R. (1969). *Cerebral organization of conscious acts: A frontal lobe function.* Paper presented to the 19th International Congress of Psychology, London, England.

Luria, A. R. (1970a). The functional organization of the brain. *Scientific American, 222,* 66-78.

Luria, A. R. (1970b). *Traumatic aphasia: Its syndrome, psychology and treatment.* Paris: Mouton.

Luria, A. R. (1973). *The working brain.* New York: Basic Books.

Luria, A. R., Naydin, V. L., Tsvetkova, L. S., & Vinarskaya, E. N. (1969). Restoration of higher cortical function following local brain damage. In P. J. Vinken & G. W. Bruyn (Eds.), *Handbook of clinical neurology, 3* (pp. 368-433). New York: Wiley.

Luria, A. R., & Tsvetkova, L. S. (1964). The programming of constructive activity in local brain injuries. *Neuropsychologia, 2,* 95-107.

Lynch, W. J. (1982). The use of electronic games in cognitive rehabilitation. In L. E. Trexler (Ed.), *Cognitive rehabilitation: Conceptualization and intervention*. New York: Plenum Press.

Lynch, W. J. (1986). An update on software in cognitive rehabilitation. *Cognitive Rehabilitation, 4*(3), 2-6.

Lynch, W. J. (1989). Computer-assisted visual-perceptual training. *Journal of Head Trauma Rehabilitation, 4*(2), 75-77.

Machover, K. (1948). *Personality projection in the drawing of the human figure.* Springfield, IL: Charles C. Thomas.

Mahoney, W. J., D'Souza, B. J., Haller, J. A., Rogers, M. C., Epstein, M. H., & Freeman, J. M. (1983). Long-term outcome of children with severe head trauma and prolonged coma. *Pediatrics, 71*, 755-762.

Malone, R. L. (1977). Expressed attitudes of families of aphasics. In J. Stubbins (Ed.), *Social and psychological aspects of disability: A handbook for practitioners.* Baltimore: University Park Press.

Mandleberg, I. A., & Brooks, D. N. (1975). Cognitive recovery after severe head injury: Serial testing on the WAIS. *Journal of Neurology, Neurosurgery, and Psychiatry, 38*, 1121-1126.

Margulis, A. R., & Fisher, M. R. (1985). Present clinical status of magnetic resonance imaging. *Magnetic Resonance Medicine, 2*, 309-327.

Marshall, L. F., & Marshall, S. B. (1985). Epidemiological and descriptive studies: Part II. Current clinical head injury research in the U.S. In D. Becker & J. T. Povlishock (Eds.), *Central nervous system trauma: Status report* (pp. 45-53). Bethesda, MD: National Institutes of Health, National Institute of Neurological and Communicative Disorders and Stroke.

Marshall, R. C. (1989). Evaluation of communication deficits of closed head injury patients. In M. D. Lezak (Ed.), *Assessment of the behavioral consequences of head trauma* (pp. 87-112). New York: Alan R. Liss.

Matarazzo, J. D. (1972). *Wechsler's measurement and appraisal of adult intelligence* (5th ed.). Baltimore: Williams & Wilkins.

Mateer, C. A., & Ruff, R. M. (1990). Effectiveness of behavior management procedures in the rehabilitation of head-injured patients. In R. L. Wood (Ed.), *Neurobehavioral sequelae of traumatic brain injury* (pp. 277-304). New York: Taylor & Frances.

Matthews, C. G., & Klove, H. (1964). *Instruction manual for the Adult Neuropsychology Test Battery.* Madison, WI: University of Wisconsin Medical School.

Matthews, D. A., Cotman, C., & Lynch, G. (1976). An electron microscopic study of lesion-induced synaptogenesis in the dentate gyrus of the adult rat: Magnitude and time cause of degeneration. *Brain Research, 115*, 11-21.

Maxwell, M., Karacostas, D., Ellenbogen, R., Brezezinski, A., Zervas, N., & Black, P. (1990). Precocious puberty following head injury. *Journal of Neurosurgery, 73*(1), 123-129.

McFie, J. (1961). The effects of hemispherectomy on intellectual functioning in cases of infantile hemiplegia. *Journal of Neurology, Neurosurgery, and Psychiatry, 24*, 240-249.

References

McFie, J. (1975). *Assessment of organic impairment*. London: Academic Press.

McGlone, J. (1978). Sex differences in functional brain asymmetry. *Cortex, 14,* 122-128.

McKay, S., & Golden, C. J. (1979). Empirical deviation of neuropsychological scales for lateralization of brain damage using the Luria-Nebraska Neuropsychological Test Battery. *Clinical Neurospychology, 1,* 1-5.

McKinlay, W. W., Brooks, D. N., & Bond, M. R. (1981). The short-term outcome of severe blunt head injury as reported by relatives of the injured person. *Journal of Neurology, Neurosurgery, and Psychiatry, 44,* 527.

Meichenbaum, D. (1977). *Cognitive behavior modification: An integrative approach*. New York: Plenum Press.

Meichenbaum, D., & Goodman, J. (1971). Training impulsive children to talk to themselves: A means of developing self-control. *Journal of Abnormal Child Psychology, 77,* 115-126.

Meirowsky, A. M. (1984). *Penetrating craniocerebral trauma*. Springfield, IL: Charles C. Thomas.

Mercer, J. R., & Lewis, J. F. (1978). *Adaptive Behavior Inventory for Children*. San Antonio: The Psychological Corporation.

Miller, E. (1984). *Recovery and management of neuropsychological impairments*. New York: Wiley.

Miller, J. D. (1983). Early evaluation and management. In M. Rosenthal, E. R. Griffith, M. Bond, & J. D. Miller (Eds.), *Rehabilitation of the head injured adult* (pp. 37-58). Philadelphia: F. A. Davis.

Miller, J. D., Butterworth, J.F., Gudeman, S. K., Faulkner, J. E., Choi, S. C., Selhorst, J. B., Harbison, J. W., Lutz, H. A., Young, H. F., & Becker, D. P. (1981). Further experience in the management of severe head injury. *Journal of Neurosurgery, 54,* 289-299.

Milner, B. (1974). Sparing of language functions after early unilateral brain damage. *Neurosciences Research Program Bulletin, 12,* 213-217.

Milner, B. (1975). Psychological aspects of focal epilepsy and its neurological management. In D. P. Purpura, J. K. Penry, & R. D. Walter (Eds.), *Advances in neurology* (pp. 299-312). New York: Raven Press.

Minuchin, S. (1974). *Families and family therapy*. Cambridge, MA: Harvard University Press.

Molnar, G. E., Jane, C. S., & Perrin, M. D. (1983). Rehabilitation of the child with head injury. In K. Shapiro (Ed.), *Pediatric head trauma* (pp. 241-271). New York: Futura.

Money, J. (1976). *A Standardized Road Map Test of Direction Sense*. San Rafael, CA: Academic Therapy Publications.

Moore, R. Y. (1974). Central regeneration and recovery of function: The problem of collateral reinervation. In D. G. Stein, J. D. Rosen, & N. Butters (Eds.), *Plasticity and recovery of function in the central nervous system* (pp. 111-129). New York: Academic Press.

245

Moyer, S. (1979). Rehabilitation of alexia: A case study. *Cortex, 15,* 139-144.

Muir, C. A., Haffey, W. J., Ott, K. J., Karaica, D., Muir, J. H., & Sutko, M. (1983). Treatment of behavioral deficits. In M. Rosenthal, E. R. Griffith, M. Bond, & J. D. Miller (Eds.), *Rehabilitation of the head injured adult* (pp. 381-384). Philadelphia: F. A. Davis.

Musante, S. E. (1983, Spring). Issues relevant to the vocational evaluation of traumatically head injured clients. *Vocational Evaluation and Work Adjustment Bulletin, 16*(2), pp. 45, 68.

Mysiw, J. W., & Jackson, R. D. (1987). Tricyclic antidepressant therapy after traumatic brain injury. *Journal of Head Trauma Rehabilitation, 2*(4), 34-42.

Naglieri, J. A. (1985). *Matrix Analogies Test.* San Antonio: The Psychological Corporation.

Narayan, R. K., Greenberg, R. P., Miller, J. D., & Enas, G. G. (1981). Improved confidence of outcome in severe head injury. *Journal of Neurosurgery, 54,* 751-762.

Narayan, R. K., Kishore, P. R., & Becker, D. P. (1982). Intracranial pressure: To monitor or not to monitor; a review of our experience with severe head injury. *Journal of Neurosurgery, 56,* 650-659.

National Head Injury Foundation. (1980). *The silent epidemic.* Framingham, MA: Author.

National Head Injury Foundation. (1982). *Coma: Its treatment and consequences.* Framingham, MA: Author.

National Head Injury Foundation. (1984). *Head injury: Hope through research.* Framingham, MA: Author.

National Head Injury Foundation. (1985). *An educator's manual: What educators need to know about students with traumatic head injury.* Framingham, MA: Author.

National Head Injury Foundation. (1988). *An educator's manual: What educators need to know about students with traumatic head injury.* Framingham, MA: Author.

National Institute of Neurological and Communicative Disorder and Stroke. (1980). *The National Head and Spinal Cord Inquiry Survey.* Bethesda, MD: Office of Scientific and Health Reports.

National Institutes of Health. (1982). Computed tomographic scanning of the brain. *Consensus Development Conference Summary, 4*(2). Washington, DC: U.S. Government Printing Office.

Naugle, R. I. (1990). Epidemiology of traumatic brain injury in adults. In E. D. Bigler (Ed.), *Traumatic brain injury: Mechanisms of damage, assessment, intervention, and outcome* (pp. 69-103). Austin: Pro-Ed.

Nelson, W. M., Finch, A. J., & Hooke, J. F. (1975). Effects of reinforcement and response-cost on the cognitive style of emotionally disturbed boys. *Journal of Abnormal Psychology, 84,* 426-428.

Newcombe, F. (1969). *Missile wounds of the brain: A study of psychological deficits.* New York: Oxford University Press.

Newcombe, F. (1981). The psychological consequences of closed head injury: Assessment and rehabilitation. *Injury, 14,* 111-136.

References

Noble, J. H., Conley, R. W., Laski, F., & Noble, M. A. (1990). Issues and problems in the treatment of traumatic brain injury. *Journal of Disability Policy Studies, 1*(2), 1-27.

North, B. (1984). *Jamieson's first notebook of head injury* (3rd ed.). London: Butterworths.

Oddy, M., & Humphrey, M. (1980). Social recovery during the year following head injury. *Journal of Neurology, Neurosurgery, and Psychiatry, 43,* 798-802.

Oddy, M., Humphrey, M., & Uttley, D. (1978a). Stresses upon relatives of head-injured patients. *British Journal of Psychiatry, 133,* 507-513.

Oddy, M., Humphrey, M., & Uttley, D. (1978b). Subjective impairment and social recovery after closed head injury. *Journal of Neurology, Neurosurgery, and Psychiatry, 41,* 611-616.

Olson, D. A. (1983). *A manual of behavioral management strategies for traumatically brain injured adults.* Chicago, IL: Northwestern University Medical School.

O'Shanick, G. J. (1987). Clinical aspects of psychopharmacologic treatment in head-injured patients. *Journal of Head Trauma Rehabilitation, 2*(4), 59-68.

Overall, J. E., & Gorham, D. R. (1962). The Brief Psychiatric Rating Scale. *Psychological Reports, 10,* 799-812.

Overs, R. P., & Healy, J. R. (1973). Stroke patients: Their spouses, families and the community. In A. B. Cobb (Ed.), *Medical and psychological aspects of disability* (pp. 87-118). Springfield, IL: Charles C. Thomas.

Paivio, A. (1971). *Imagery and verbal responses.* New York: Holt, Rinehart, & Winston.

Pang, D. (1985). Pathophysiologic correlations of neurobehavioral syndromes following closed head injury. In M. Ylvisaker (Ed.), *Head injury rehabilitation: Children and adolescents* (pp. 3-71). San Diego: College-Hill Press.

Parente, R., & Anderson-Parente, J. K. (1989). Retraining memory: Theory and applications. *Head Trauma Rehabilitation, 4*(3), 55-65.

Parker, R. S. (1990). *Traumatic brain injury and neuropsychological impairment: Sensorimotor, cognitive, emotional and adaptive problems of children and adults.* New York: Springer-Verlag.

Parmelee, D., & O'Shanick, G. J. (1987). Neuropsychiatric interventions with head injured children and adolescents. *Brain Injury, 1*(1), 41-47.

Patten, B. M. (1972). The ancient art of memory. *Archives of Neurology, 26,* 25.

Patten, B. M. (1982). *Modality specific memory disorders.* New York: Neurological Institute.

Peck, A. W., Stern, W. C., & Watkinson, C. (1983). Incidence of seizures during treatment with tricyclic antidepressant drugs and bupropion. *Journal of Clinical Psychiatry, 44,* 197-201.

Piaget, J. (1969). *The child's conception of the world.* Patterson, NJ: Littlefield, Adams.

Polinko, P. R. (1985). Working with the family: The acute phase. In M. Ylvisaker (Ed.), *Head injury rehabilitation: Children and adolescents* (pp. 91-115). San Diego: College-Hill Press.

Porch, B. E. (1967). *Porch Index of Communicative Ability.* Palo Alto, CA: Consulting Psychologists Press.

Porteus, S. D. (1959). *The Maze Test and clinical psychology.* Palo Alto, CA: Pacific Books.

Porteus, S. D. (1965). *Porteus Mazes.* San Antonio: The Psychological Corporation.

Prigatano, G. P. (1991). Disordered mind, wounded soul: The emerging role of psychotherapy in rehabilitation after brain injury. *Journal of Head Trauma Rehabilitation, 6*(4), 1-10.

Prigatano, G. P., Pepping, M., & Klonoff, P. (1986). Cognitive, personality, and psychosocial factors in the neuropsychological assessment of brain-injured patients. In B. Uzzell & Y. Gross (Eds.), *Clinical neuropsychology of intervention* (pp. 135-167). Boston: Martinus Nijhoff.

Purdue Research Foundation. (1948). *Examiner's manual for the Purdue Pegboard.* Chicago: Science Research Associates.

Quay, H. C., & Peterson, D. R. (1983). *Revised Behavior Problem Checklist.* Coral Gables, FL: University of Miami.

Raimondi, A. J., & Hirschauer, J. (1984). Head injury in the infant and toddler. *Child's Brain, 11*, 12-35.

Ransohoff, J., & Koslow, M. (1978). Guide to the diagnosis and management of cerebral injury. *Hospital Medicine, 5,* 127-143.

Raven, J. C. (1986). *Guide to the Standard Progressive Matrices.* San Antonio: The Psychological Corporation.

Raven, J. C. (1986). *Guide to using the Coloured Progressive Matrices.* San Antonio: The Psychological Corporation.

Redford, J. (Ed.). (1980). *Orthotics Etc.* Baltimore: Williams & Wilkins.

Reitan, R. M. (1955). Certain undifferential effects of left and right cerebral lesions in human adults. *Journal of Comparative Physiology Psychology, 48,* 474-477.

Reitan, R. M. (1959). *Manual for administration of neuropsychological test batteries for adults and children.* Unpublished manual, Indiana University Medical Center, Indianapolis.

Reitan, R. M. (1968). Psychological assessment of deficits associated with brain lesions in subjects with normal and subnormal intelligence. In J. L. Khanna (Ed.), *Brain damage and mental retardation: A psychological evaluation* (pp. 44-94). Springfield, IL: Charles C. Thomas.

Reitan, R. M., & Davison, L. A. (1974). *Clinical neuropsychology: Current status and applications.* New York: Wiley.

Reynolds, C. (1981). The neuropsychological basis of intelligence. In G. W. Hynd & J. E. Obrzut (Eds.), *Neuropsychological assessment and the school-aged child: Issues and procedures* (pp. 87-124). New York: Grune & Stratton.

Richardson, F. (1963). Some effects of severe head injury. *Developmental Medicine and Child Neurology, 5,* 471-482.

Richman, S., & Gholson, B. (1978). Strategy modeling, age and information-processing efficiency. *Journal of Experimental Psychology, 26,* 58-70.

References

Rimel, R. W., Giordani, B., Barth, J. T., Boll, T. J., & Jane, J. A. (1981). Disability caused by minor head injury. *Neurosurgery, 9,* 221-228.

Rimel, R., Giordani, B., Barth, J., & Jane, J. (1982). Moderate head injury: Completing the clinical spectrum of brain trauma. *Neurosurgery, 11,* 344-351.

Ritvo, E. R., Ornitz, E. M., & Walter, R. D. (1970). Correlation of psychiatric diagnosis and EEG findings: A double-blind study of 184 hospitalized children. *American Journal of Psychiatry, 126,* 988-996.

Roach, E. G., & Kephart, N. C. (1966). *Purdue Perceptual-Motor Survey.* San Antonio: The Psychological Corporation.

Roberts, G. E., & McArthur, D. S. (1982). *Roberts Apperception Test.* Los Angeles, CA: Western Psychological Services.

Robinson, H. B., & Robinson, N. M. (1965). *The mentally retarded child: A psychological approach.* New York: McGraw Hill.

Rollin, W. J. (1984). Family therapy with the aphasic adult. In J. Eisenson (Ed.), *Adult aphasia* (pp. 252-282). Englewood Cliffs, NJ: Prentice-Hall.

Rorschach, H. (1945). *Rorschach technique.* San Antonio: The Psychological Corporation.

Rosen, C. D., & Gerring, J. P. (1986). *Head trauma: Educational reintegration.* San Diego: College-Hill Press.

Rosenthal, M., Griffith, E. R., Bond, M. R., & Miller, J. D. (Eds.). (1983). *Rehabilitation of the head injured adult.* Philadelphia: F. A. Davis.

Rosenthal, M., & Muir, C. (1983). Methods of family intervention. In M. Rosenthal, E. Griffith, M. Bond, & J. D. Miller (Eds.), *Rehabilitation of the head injured adult* (pp. 407-419). Philadelphia: F. A. Davis.

Rosner, B. S. (1974). Recovery of function and localization of function in historical perspective. In D. G. Stein, J. J. Rosen, & N. Butters (Eds.), *Plasticity and recovery of function in the central nervous system* (pp. 1-31). New York: Academic Press.

Rourke, B. P. (1983). Reading and spelling disabilities: A developmental neuropsychological perspective. In U. Kirk (Ed.), *Neuropsychology of language, reading, and spelling.* New York: Academic Press.

Rourke, B. P., Bakker, D. J., Fisk, J. L., & Strang, J. D. (1983). *Child neuropsychology: An introduction to theory, research, and clinical practice.* New York: Guilford Press.

Rourke, B. P., & Gates, R. D. (1980). *Underlining Test Preliminary Norms.* Windsor, Ontario: Authors.

Rubens, A. (1977). The role of changes in the central nervous system during recovery from aphasia. *Rationale for adult aphasia therapy* (pp. 28-43). Lincoln, NB: University of Nebraska Press.

Rudel, R. G. (1978). Neuroplasticity: Implications for development and education. In J. S. Chall & A. F. Mirsky (Eds.), *Education and the brain, Part II.* Chicago: University of Chicago Press.

Rudel, R. G., Teuber, H. L., & Twitchell, T. E. (1974). Levels of impairment of sensory-motor functions in children with early brain damage. *Neuropsychologia, 12,* 95-108.

Rusch, M. D., Grunert, B. K., Erdmann, B. R., & Lynch, N. T. (1980). *Cognitive retraining of brain-injured adults.* Milwaukee, WI: Curative Rehabilitation Center.

Russell, E. W. (1984). Theory and development of pattern analysis methods related to the Halstead-Reitan Battery. In P. E. Logue & T. M. Shear (Eds.), *Clinical neuropsychology.* Springfield, IL: Charles C. Thomas.

Russell, E. W., Neuringer, C., & Goldstein, G. (1970). *Assessment of brain damage.* New York: Wiley.

Russell, W. R. (1932). Cerebral involvement in head injury. A study based on the examination of 200 cases. *Brain, 55,* 549-603.

Russell, W. R. (1971). *The traumatic amnesias.* London: Oxford University Press.

Rutter, M. (1981). Psychological sequelae of brain damage in children. *American Journal of Psychiatry, 138,* 1533-1544.

Rutter, M., Chadwick, O., & Shaffer, D. (1983). Head injury. In M. Rutter (Ed.), *Developmental neuropsychiatry* (pp. 83-111). New York: Guilford Press.

Rutter, M., Graham, P., & Yule, W. (1970). *A neuropsychiatric study in childhood.* London: Spastics International Medical Publications/Heinemann Medical Books.

Salter, A. (1961). *Conditioned reflex therapy.* New York: Putnam Press.

Sand, P. L., Trieschman, R. B., Fordyce, W. E., & Fowler, R. S. (1970). Behavior modification in the medical rehabilitation setting: Rationale and some applications. *Rehabilitation Research Practice Review, 1,* 11.

Sarno, M. T. (1980). The nature of verbal impairment after closed head injury. *Journal of Nervous and Mental Disease, 168,* 685-692.

Sarno, M. T. (1984). Verbal impairment after closed head injury: Report of a replication study. *Journal of Nervous and Mental Disease, 172,* 475-479.

Sarno, M. T., & Levin, H. S. (1985). *Speech and language evaluation in neurology.* Available from National Institute of Handicapped Research, Washington, DC.

Sattler, J. M. (1982). *Assessment of children's intelligence and special abilities* (2nd ed.). Boston: Allyn & Bacon.

Sattler, J. M. (1988). *Assessment of children* (3rd ed.). San Diego: Author.

Savage, R. (1991). Identification, classification, and placement of traumatically brain-injured students. *Journal of Head Trauma Rehabilitation, 6*(1), 1-9.

Savage, R. C., & Carter, R. (1984, Nov/Dec). Re-entry: The head injured student returns to school. *Cognitive Rehabilitation,* pp. 28-33.

Schaefer, C., & O'Connor, K. (1983). *Handbook of play therapy.* New York: Wiley.

Schmidt, N., & Lynch, N. (1983, Winter). Ask the experts. *National Head Injury Foundation Newsletter, 3* (2).

Schneider, G. E. (1979). Is it really better to have your brain lesion early? A revision of the Kennard principle. *Neuropsychologia, 17,* 557-583.

Schuell, H., Jenkins, J., & Jimenez-Pabon, E. (1964). *Aphasia in adults.* New York: Harper & Row.

References

Scott, E. P., Hatten, P. H., & Jan, J. E. (1979). Educational and vocational training of blind and partially sighted children in Canada and the U.S. *Clinics Developmental Medicine, 73,* 156-165.

Segalowitz, S. J., & Gruber, F. A. (Eds.). (1977). *Language development and neurological theory.* New York: Academic Press.

Seidel, V. P., Chadwick, O., & Rutter, M. (1975). Psychological disorders in crippled children: A comparative study of children with and without brain damage. *Developmental Medicine and Child Neurology, 17,* 563-573.

Selz, M. (1981). Halstead-Reitan neuropsychological test batteries for children. In W. Hynd & J. E. Obrzut (Eds.), *Neuropsychological assessment and the school-aged child: Issues and procedures* (pp. 195-236). New York: Grune & Stratton.

Shaffer, D., Bijur, P., Chadwick, O., & Rutter, M. (1980). Head injury and later reading disability. *Journal of the American Academy of Child Psychiatry, 19,* 592-610.

Shaffer, D., Chadwick, O., & Rutter, M. (1975). Psychiatric outcome of localized head injury in children: *Ciba Foundation Symposium, 34,* (new series).

Shapiro, K. (1983). Care and evaluation of the conscious head-injured child. In K. Shapiro (Ed.), *Pediatric head trauma* (pp. 11-26). New York: Futura.

Shapiro, K. (1985). Head injury in children. D. Becker & J. T. Povlishock (Eds.), *Central nervous system trauma: Status report* (pp. 243-255). Bethesda, MD: National Institutes of Health, National Institute of Neurological and Communicative Disorders and Stroke.

Silver, S. M., & Kay, T. (1989). Closed head trauma: Vocational assessment. In M. Lezak (Ed.), *Assessment of the behavioral consequences of head trauma* (pp. 171-194). New York: Alan Liss.

Sims, A. C. (1985). Head injury, neurosis, and accident proneness. *Advances in Psychosomatic Medicine, 13,* 49-70.

Sine, R. D., Liss, S. E., Rousch, R. E., & Holcomb, J. D. (Eds.). (1977). *Basic rehabilitation techniques: A self-instructional guide.* Germantown, MD: Aspen Systems.

Singer, H. S., & Freeman, J. M. (1978). Head trauma for the pediatrician. *Pediatrics, 62*(5), 819-825.

Skelly, M. (1979). *Amer-Ind gestural code based on universal American Indian hand talk.* New York: Elsevier.

Slenkovich, J. E. (1987, February). Extended school: When is it really required? *School's advocate,* pp. 65-71.

Smith, A. (1971). Objective indices of severity of chronic aphasia of stroke patients. *Journal of Speech and Hearing Disorders, 36,* 167-207.

Smith, A. (1975). Neuropsychological testing in neurological disorders. In W. J. Friedlander (Ed.), *Advances in neurology* (Vol. 7). New York: Raven Press.

Smith, D. B. (1990). Antiepileptic drug selection in adults. In D. B. Smith (Ed.), *Epilepsy: Current approaches to diagnosis and treatment* (pp. 111-139). New York: Raven Press.

Smith, G. J., & Ylvisaker, M. (1985). Cognitive rehabilitation therapy: Early stages of recovery. In M. Ylvisaker (Ed.), *Head injury rehabilitation: Children and adolescents* (pp. 275-287). San Diego: College-Hill Press.

Smith, R. K. (1983). Prevocational programming in the rehabilitation of the head-injured patient. *Journal of the American Physical Therapy Association, 63,* 2026-2029.

Sohlberg, M. M., & Mateer, C. A. (1989). *Introduction to cognitive rehabilitation: Theory and practice.* New York: Guilford Press.

Sosin, D. M., Sacks, J. J., & Smith, S. (1989). Head injury—associated deaths in the United States. *Journal of the American Medical Association, 262*(16), 2251-2255.

Sparks, R., Helm, N., & Albert, M. (1974). Aphasia rehabilitation resulting from melodic intonation therapy. *Cortex, 10,* 303-316.

Sparrow, S., Balla, D. A., & Cicchetti, D. V. (1984). *Vineland Adaptive Behavior Scales.* Circle Pines, MN: American Guidance Service.

Spivack, G., & Spotts, J. (1966). *Devereux Child Behavior Rating Scale manual.* Devon, PA: Devereux Foundation.

Stern, J. M. (1985). The quality of the psychotherapeutic process in brain-injured patients. *Scandinavian Journal of Rehabilitative Medicine, 12,* 42-43.

Stover, S. L., & Zeiger, H. E. (1976). Head injury in teenagers: Functional recovery correlated with duration of coma. *Archives of Physical Medicine and Rehabilitation, 57,* 201-205.

Strang, J. D. (1983). *Similarities between Piaget's theory of intellectual development (sensorimotor period) and early brain development.* Prepublication manuscript, University of Windsor.

Strich, S. J. (1969). The pathology of brain damage due to blunt head injuries. In A. E. Walker. W. F. Caveness, & M. Critchley (Eds.), *The late effects of head injury.* Springfield, IL: Charles C. Thomas.

Strich, S. J. (1970). Lesions in the cerebral hemispheres after blunt head injury. In S. Sesvitt & H. B. Stoner (Eds.), *The pathology of trauma* (pp. 166-171). London: BMA House.

Sutton, R. L., Weaver, M. S., & Feeney, D. F. (1987). Drug-induced modifications of behavioral recovery following cortical trauma. *Journal of Head Trauma Rehabilitation, 2*(4), 50-58.

Symonds, C. P. (1940). Concussion and contusion of the brain and their sequelae. In S. Brock (Ed.), *Injuries of the skull, brain and spinal cord* (pp. 69-111). Baltimore: Williams & Wilkins.

Symonds, C. P. (1962). Concussion and its sequelae. *Lancet, i,* 1-5.

Szekeres, S., Ylvisaker, M., & Holland, A. (1985). Cognitive rehabilitation therapy: A framework for intervention. In M. Ylvisaker (Ed.), *Head injury rehabilitation: Children and adolescents* (pp. 219-247). San Diego: College-Hill Press.

Tabaddor, K. (1982). Emergency care; initial evaluation. In P. Cooper (Ed.), *Head injury* (pp. 15-27). Baltimore: Williams & Wilkins.

References

Tarnow, J. D. (1984). Pediatric and adolescent patients in rehabilitation. In D. W. Krueger (Ed.), *Emotional rehabilitation of physical trauma and disability* (pp. 63-78). New York: SP Medical & Scientific Books.

Tarter, R. E., & Edwards, K. L. (1986). Neuropsychological batteries. In T. Incagnoli, G. Goldstein, & C. J. Golden (Eds.), *Clinical application of neuropsychological test batteries* (pp. 135-153). New York: Plenum Press.

Taylor, G. P., & Persons, R. W. (1970). Behavior modification techniques in a physical medicine and rehabilitation center. *Journal of Psychology, 74,* 117.

Taylor, M. T. (1964). Language therapy. In H. G. Burr (Ed.), *The aphasic adult: Evaluation rehabilitation.* Charlottesville, VA: Wayside Press.

Teasdale, G., & Jennett, B. (1974). Assessment of coma and impaired consciousness: A practical scale. *Lancet, ii,* 81-84.

Teasdale, G., & Jennett, B. (1976). Assessment and prognosis of coma after head injury. *Acta Neurochir, 34,* 45-55.

Telzrow, C. (1987). Management of academic and educational problems in head injury. *Journal of Learning Disabilities, 20*(9), 536-545.

Teuber, H. L. (1974). Recovery of function after lesions of the central nervous system: History and prospects. *Neurosciences Research Program Bulletin, 12,* 197-213.

Thompsen, I. V. (1974). The patient with severe head injury and his family. *Scandinavian Journal of Rehabilitative Medicine, 6,* 180-183.

Thompsen, I. V. (1975). Evaluation and outcome of aphasia in patients with severe closed head injury. *Journal of Neurosurgery and Psychiatry, 38,* 713-718.

Thorndike, R. L., Hagen, E. P., & Sattler, J. M. (1986). *Stanford-Binet Intelligence Scale: Fourth Edition.* Chicago: Riverside Publishing.

Tufts Medical Center. (1984). *Psychological and vocational aspects of head injury: Training course for MRC.* (Tufts Medical Rehabilitation Research and Training Center). Boston, MA: Author.

Ungerstedt, V. (1971). Post synaptic supersensitivity after 6-hydroxy-dopamine induced degeneration of nigro-striatal dopamine system. *Acta Physiologica Scandinavica, 367,* 69-93.

University of Virginia Medical Center. (1988). *First aid in seizure care.* Available from Blue Ridge Hospital, Epilepsy Unit, 1 West, Charlottesville, VA 22901.

Urdang, L., & Swallow, H. H. (Eds.). (1983). *Mosby's medical and nursing dictionary.* London: C. V. Mosby.

U.S. Department of Health, Education, and Welfare. (1979). *Aphasia: Hope through research.* (National Institutes of Health, Publication No. 80-391). Washington, DC: U.S. Government Printing Office.

Varney, N. R., & Benton, A. L. (1979). Phonemic discrimination in aural comprehension among aphasic patients. *Journal of Clinical Neuropsychology, 1,* 65-73.

Varney, N. R., & Benton, A. L. (1982). Qualitative aspects of pantomine recognition defect in aphasia. *Brain and Cognition, 1,* 132-139.

Von Monakow, C. (1914). *Die Lokalisation im Grosshirn und der Abbau. Der Funktion durch Kortikale Herde.* Wiesbaden: J. F. Bergmann.

Walker, K. F. (1989). Clinically relevant features of the visual system. *Journal of Head Trauma Rehabilitation, 4*(2), 1-8.

Walsh, K. W. (1978). *Neuropsychology: A clinical approach.* Edinburgh: Churchill-Livingstone.

Walton, R. (1982). Lecithin and physostigmine for posttraumatic memory and cognitive deficits. *Psychosomatics, 23,* 435-436.

Wang, M. C., Reynolds, M. C., & Schwartz, L. L. (1989). Adaptive instruction: An alternative educational approach for students with special needs. In J. Graden, J. Zins, & M. Curtis (Eds.), *Alternative educational delivery systems* (pp. 199-220). Washington, DC: NASP.

Wechsler, D. (1981). *Wechsler Adult Intelligence Scale - Revised.* San Antonio: The Psychological Corporation.

Wechsler, D. (1987). *Wechsler Memory Scale - Revised.* San Antonio, TX: The Psychological Corporation.

Wechsler, D. (1989). *Wechsler Preschool and Primary Scale of Intelligence - Revised.* San Antonio: The Psychological Corporation.

Wechsler, D. (1991). *Wechsler Intelligence Scale for Children-III.* San Antonio: The Psychological Corporation.

Weddell, R., Oddy, M., & Jenkins, D. (1980). Social adjustment after rehabilitation: A two-year follow-up of patients with severe head injury. *Psychological Medicine, 10,* 257-263.

Weinstein, E. A., & Lyerly, O. G. (1968). Confabulation following brain injury. *Archives of General Psychiatry, 18,* 348-354.

Weinstein, G. S., & Wells, C. E. (1981). Case studies in neuropsychiatry: Post-traumatic psychiatric dysfunction; Diagnosis and treatment. *Clinical Psychiatry, 42,* 120-122.

Weniger, D., Huber, W., Stachowiak, F. J., & Poeck, K. (1980). Treatment of aphasia on a linguistic basis. In M. T. Sarno & O. Hook (Eds.), *Aphasia: Assessment and treatment.* Stockholm: Almquist & Wiksell.

Wepman, J. M. (1951). *Recovery from aphasia.* New York: Ronald Press.

Wepman, J. (1968). The modality concept. In H. K. Smith (Ed.), *Perception and reading.* Newark, DE: International Reading Association.

Wepman, J. M., & Turaids, D. (1975). *Spatial Orientation Memory Test. Manual of Directions.* Palm Springs, CA: Language Research Associates.

West, D. R., Deadwyler, S. A., Cotman, C. W., & Lynch, G. S. (1976). An experimental test of diaschisis. *Behavioral Biology, 22,* 419-425.

Westervelt, V., & Rozzi, F. (1985, March). *Social skills training: Interpersonal process recall for head injured children and adolescents.* Paper presented at the Children's Rehabilitation Center, University of Virginia Medical Center, Charlottesville, VA.

References

Willer, B., Abosch, S., & Dahmer, E. (1990). Epidemiology of disability from traumatic brain injury. In R. L. Wood (Ed.), *Neurobehavioral sequelae of traumatic brain injury* (pp. 18-33). London: Taylor and Frances.

Williams, J. R., Csongradi, J. J., & LeBlanc, M. A. (1982). *A guide to controls: Selection, mounting, and application.* Palo Alto, CA: Children's Hospital at Stanford.

Wilson, B., Cockburn, J., & Baddeley, A. (1985). *Rivermead Behavioral Memory Test.* Gaylord, MI: National Rehabilitation Services.

Wilson, B. A. (1987). *Rehabilitation of memory.* New York: Guilford Press.

Wilson, B. A., & Moffat, N. (1984). *Clinical management of memory problems.* Rockville, MD: Aspen.

Wilson, R. S., Rosenbaum, G., & Brown, G. (1979). The problem of premorbid intelligence in neuropsychological assessment. *Journal of Clinical Neuropsychology, 1,* 49-54.

Wirt, R. D., Lachar, D., Klinedinst, J. K., & Seat, P. D. (1977). *Multidimensional description of child personality. A manual for the Personality Inventory of Children.* Los Angeles: Western Psychological Services.

Wood, R. L. (1987). *Brain injury rehabilitation: A neurobehavioral approach.* Rockville, MD: Aspen.

Wood, R. L. (1990a). Conditioning procedures in brain injury rehabilitation. In R. L. Wood (Ed.), *Neurobehavioral sequelae of traumatic brain injury* (pp. 153-174). New York: Taylor & Frances.

Wood, R. L. (1990b). Neurobehavioral paradigm for brain injury rehabilitation. In R. Wood (Ed.), *Neurobehavioral sequelae of traumatic brain injury* (pp. 3-17). New York: Taylor & Frances.

Wood, R. L. (1991). Critical analysis of the concept of sensory stimulation for patients in vegetative states. *Brain Injury, 9*(4), 401-409.

Wood, R. L., & Eames, P. (1981). Application of behavior modification in the rehabilitation of traumatically brain-injured patients. In G. Davey (Ed.), *Applications of conditioning theory* (pp. 81-101). London: Methuen.

Woodcock, R. W., & Johnson, M. B. (1989). *Woodcock-Johnson Psycho-Educational Battery—Revised.* Allen, TX: DLM.

Woods, B. T. (1980). The restricted effects of right-hemisphere lesions after age one: Wechsler test data. *Neuropsychologia, 18,* 65-70.

World Health Organization. (1975). *The International Classification of Diseases, Vol. 1, Diseases. Tabular List.* Ann Arbor: Edwards Brothers, Inc.

Ylvisaker, M. (Ed.). (1985). *Head injury rehabilitation: Children and adolescents.* San Diego: College-Hill Press.

Ylvisaker, M., Hartwick, P., & Stevens, M. (1991). School re-entry following head injury: Managing transition from hospital to school. *Journal of Head Trauma Rehabilitation, 6*(1), 10-22.

Yokota, H., Kurokawa, A., Otsuka, T., Kobayashi, S., & Nakazawa, S. (1991). Significance of magnetic resonance imaging in acute head injury. *Journal of Trauma, 31*(3), 351-357.

255

Zarski, J. J., DePompei, R., West, J. D., & Hall, D. E. (1988). Chronic illness: Stressors, the adjustment process and family focused interventions. *Journal of Mental Health Counseling, 10*(2), 145-158.

SUBJECT INDEX